THE
Make-Up Center
BOOK

THE
Make-Up Center
BOOK

CARYL WENDKOS-LA TORRE

St. Martin's Press
NEW YORK

To and because of The White Bow, without whom I'd never have translated painting a face to cosmetics!

And to Brad, Gina, and Angela who think I'm special, not because I actually am but because they are!

Copyright © 1979 by Caryl Wendkos-La Torre.
All rights reserved. For information, write:
St. Martin's Press, Inc., 175 Fifth Avenue, New York, N.Y. 10010.
Manufactured in the United States of America
Library of Congress Catalog Card Number: 78-19401

DESIGNED BY BETTY BINNS

Library of Congress Cataloging in Publication Data
Wendkos-La Torre, Caryl.
    The Make-Up Center Book.

    1. Cosmetics.   2. Make-Up Center.   I. Title.
RA778.W24   646.7'2   78-19401
ISBN 0-312-50655-4

CONTENTS

PREFACE

Before I even begin, I feel it is important to point out that this book would not be as functional if I omitted mentioning exact brand names. I would, however, like to make two things clear relative to this. First, I have absolutely no axe to grind when it comes to cosmetic products that compete with On Stage make-up, the brand we sell at the Make-Up Center. In this text I mention those that I personally feel are good — underline **personally.** I am not a chemist nor a computer, and besides there is no real measure for the worth of a product except the subjective one. The products I have found to be successful—by using them personally and applying them to others—may not necessarily react 100 percent the same on everyone. That is why I continue to stress the importance of testing for yourself! You may find some of your favorite products listed in this book, or you may not. That does not mean, however, that those left unlisted are inferior in quality or performance. It simply means that either I did not like them or I was unfamiliar with them. I do not represent myself as a cosmetic products mavin, only (and humbleness be damned) an expert of the what-to-do-with-them species.

The second and most obvious point to be cleared is my active involvement with Make-Up Center and the delicate position that puts me in relative to the specific mention of products. The purpose of this book is not to sell cosmetics. The purpose is to instruct the reader in the simple and professional means of improving the appearance. It would not behoove me, however, to omit mentioning the Make-Up Center On Stage products on these grounds. As an integral part of the team that originates, designs, and conceives these products, I am in the very best position to know what sincere care, integrity, and high standards of excellence go into their conception and manufacture. Let's face it, with all the cosmetics now on the market, it would be a foolhardy, misguided move to deliberately expend time, money, and effort on merchandise that was not as good as it could possibly be. The difference between a really good product and a not so good one is a mere matter of pennies! The biggest expense is incurred in packaging, management, and marketing. In any event, you will note that On Stage is mentioned frequently. After all, it's the product that I know best. If it is not **the** best product on the market, it is as good as any and better than many!

INTRODUCTION

When Venning wrote, "Beauty is but skin deep," he must have been placating some dreary and unattractive loved one. The fact is that although he was perfectly right — beauty **is** only skin deep — there isn't a woman alive who doesn't aspire to that shallow ambition!

Since her very beginning, woman has devised and designed, conceived and concocted creams, mixtures, and lotions to effect a more beautiful image, while man has accepted, acknowledged, sponsored and endorsed this never-ending task. In fact, man has himself become so involved that his own level of vanity has become on a par with hers. And, if we are to believe that oft-used advertising header, "Only a hairdresser knows for sure," the "weaker" sex should no longer be referred to as the "fairer" sex!

Being beautiful or attractive affects men and women in every strata of life and in every humdrum facet of its living. It is an attitude that has become so much a reflex that we, unfortunately, are often guilty of discriminatory tactics. We judge people too quickly, reacting to the way they look rather than to what they have to offer. The prettier girls get the most dances, the more dates, the handsomer escorts. They get the leading roles, the quicker interviews, the more patient treatment. The plain girls are the librarians, the charwomen, the spinster teachers. It's all Hollywood, yes, but somewhere along the way we've all unconsciously accepted it!

To illustrate just how true this is, psychologist Elaine Walters and her colleagues conducted a study wherein they teamed up a group of college students for a "blind date." Each participant was judged beforehand on personality, intelligence, beauty, etc. Afterward the students were asked, one by one, if they would like to see their individual partners again. Every consideration beyond attractiveness was ignored; good looks were all that mattered!

Alas, as we grow older, we do not grow wiser. Mature people are subject to these same prejudices. In a study done by two universities, Minnesota and Wisconsin psychologists found that the Grey Panthers attributed happy marriages, high incomes, happiness, poise, and strength of character to the attractive people in a series of photographs they were asked to evaluate, while the unattractive people were generally considered deficient in these traits.

To further prove the point, let's consider the study done by Dr. Mary Lee Meiners and Dr. John Sheposh. The participants were shown one-minute videotapes of a man and a series of different women. The man was always the same one, but the women became progressively less attractive in each shot. The viewers were informed about each woman's occupation so they could judge her intelligence, poise, sociability, etc. The eighty volunteers — forty men, forty women — were then asked to evaluate the man. The exceptionally interesting result was that the more attractive the woman, the higher rating the man received.

What does it mean? Simply that a man who can attract a good-looking woman companion "must" necessarily have more on the ball than that same man when accompanied by a less attractive female!

One of the most disturbing conclusions to be reached is that brains, personality, wit, honesty, talent, or any other favorable attribute we strive to claim as part of our character doesn't matter a whit!

Something equally disturbing is the reaction of people to a "mixed" couple, a plain man and a beautiful woman or vice versa. In the case of the plain man/beautiful woman, the man is presumed to be intelligent, very gainfully employed, witty, personable, and happy. The very curious aspect is that when the plain woman, on the other hand, is accompanied by a handsome male companion, none of those same aspects is assumed. She is still just a plain woman who, of course, "must have a lot of money"! Funny how the double standard persists!

Similar studies have been made using so-called trained and educated minds. Teachers, who spend a great deal of time in

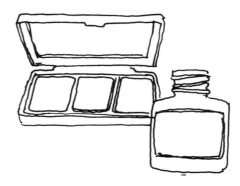

their college experience attending psychology classes and in efforts to train their minds to think objectively, were asked to evaluate report cards relative to the pupil's appearance. By and large the teachers guessed that the higher IQs belonged to the better-looking pupil. They went so far as to presume that the parents of the better-looking pupils were smarter, more interested in their children's progress, and got along better with each other.

It is obvious, then, that looking attractive is more important than just satisfying simple vanity. It affects our every living moment!

We generally **are** just exactly what we think we are. When we are secure in our attractiveness, we unconsciously project an aura of confidence, calm, and beauty. It's as easy to "read" as large print. So what? So to say that beauty is but skin deep is not exactly true. Feeling pretty makes the attitudes change, the spirits rise, the head clearer, and greater challenges are more easily accepted. Attractive people stride instead of slink; they are generally not afraid to stand up and be noticed; and they have a more open and inviting magnetism.

But, is that all there is? Of course not. A ravishing beauty can very quickly become a boring beauty, once the mouth opens and it is discovered that no one's at home. (For those of you who, nonetheless, opt for simple skin-deep beauty, consider spending the rest of your days with the type of companion who couldn't care less what's in the head department. I think it's safe to say that the majority would contend that the only thing that can actually make this type of beauty look good is distance!)

So, please don't get me wrong. I do not advocate putting all your eggs in the beauty basket. This book, however, is written solely to show you how to affect the way the observer sees you. How to redesign the bad features, clarify the neither-here-nor-there features, and spotlight (for all they're worth) the good features. How to accentuate the positive and minimize the negative.

What happens after that is up to you!

Looking beautiful is simple, really simple, once you learn the tricks. To **keep** looking that way is the real magic!

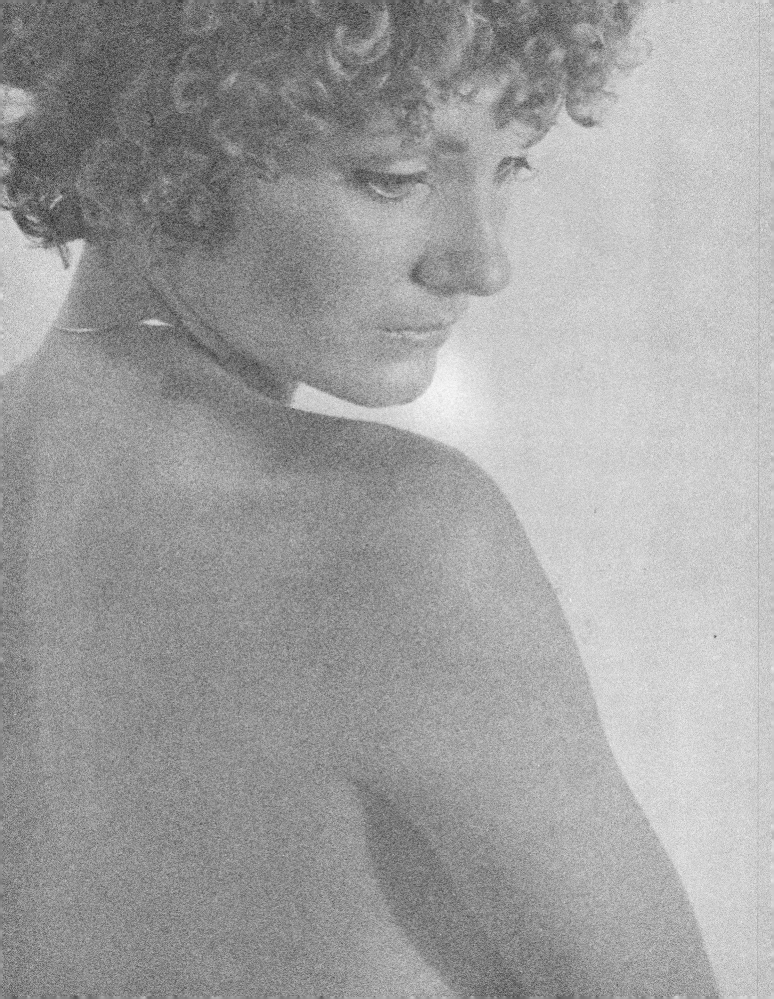

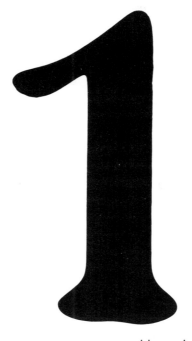

CARING FOR YOUR SKIN

As a first step in the quest for beauty you should understand the skin and the way it works. In my opinion, looking beautiful is directly related to clear, healthy skin.

Have you ever seen an acne-skinned starlet or a glamorous model with blackheads? And if you found out that your favorite movie star had pimples on his back, would he still seem as sexy?

Just as an artist must begin his work on a clean, clear canvas, so should you have the perfect background for your efforts. Unfortunately, many of us do not know how to properly care for our skins. For this reason it is important that you learn a little about it.

For instance, did you know that one square inch of skin contains: 60 hairs, 94 oil glands, 19 feet of blood vessels, 625 sweat glands, 19,000 sensory cells, 75 feet of nerves, 155 pressure receptors, 1,250 pain receptors, 12 cold receptors, 12 heat receptors, and 19,000,000 cells?

The role of the skin is to create a membrane between the delicate organisms of the body and the air. The skin protects while also maintaining the proper amount of moisture within the body. It functions as the regulating and protective system.

The skin is made up of three principal layers. These basic layers, in themselves, are made up of several layers. Plump new cells are constantly being made in the first main layer, the **epidermis.** As a result of this multiplication, the cells are continuously being pushed toward the surface. As these cells move, they undergo a series of changes until, as they reach closer to the surface, they die. These dead cells make up the ten or twenty very flat, dry layers of surface skin.

The second innermost layer of skin, the **dermis,** where the blood vessels and nerves lie, consists of fibrous materials called **collagen & elastin.** These substances are the tough elastic materials which let us change our facial expressions. We smile, we frown, we sneer, and when we are done the skin promptly returns to its original position.

As we age, the entire cycle slows down. Fewer plump cells are being formed, the dead cells adhere longer, and the elasticity of the collagen fibers tires. As the cells reduce in mass and the collagen loses its resiliency, the skin creases, wrinkles, and sags. A parallel is easily seen in the plum-to-prune metamorphosis.

Unfortunately, Ponce de Léon never found that fountain of youth, and all we can do is retard the inevitable.

For some skins, however, the inevitable comes later than for others. Oily skin is better able to maintain elasticity than dry skin. It's fairly easy to understand why. A brittle, dried leather pelt, if immersed in or constantly massaged with cream or oil, will soon recapture its flexibility.

Is the solution, then, to slather the skin with oil? Unfortunately, no. The skin must "breathe," and the tiny orifices within the skin, improperly called pores, must be kept free to excrete perspiration and the natural oil secreted by the sebaceous glands, called **sebum**. These tiny "holes" have very

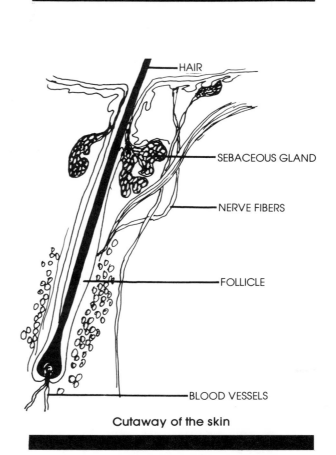

HAIR

SEBACEOUS GLAND

NERVE FIBERS

FOLLICLE

BLOOD VESSELS

Cutaway of the skin

different purposes. The duct through which sweat is excreted is the only orifice that may properly be termed a **pore**. These orifices, incidentally, are so tiny that they cannot even be detected with a magnifying glass. The correct name for what we usually call a pore is **ostium**, or **follicular orifice**. (One can see why the colloquialism has been so generally adopted!)

This tiny channel is the one that generally can be readily seen on the surface of the skin. It is the orifice through which the hair of the skin projects and wherein the sebaceous gland delivers its secretion. For purposes of maintaining a clear understanding and less confusion, the follicular orifice will improperly be designated as the pore in this text.

The first step is to diminish the wear and tear on the collagen and elastin fibers by curtailing the unattractive facial expressions to some degree. Of course that does not mean wearing a poker face — nor does it mean that, once the first line appears, you might as well start shopping for a rocker. A face that's expressive and looks as though it's alive and used to enjoying life is much more beautiful than a frozen, flawless one. To many people, flawless beauty is directly related to flawless boredom!

What it does mean, however, is that some effort should be made to break the habit of constantly moving the face into po-

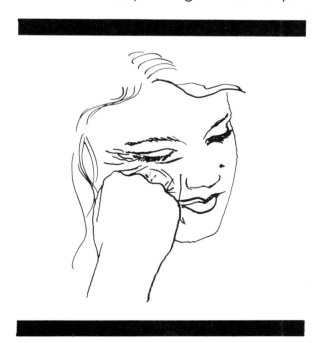

sitions that one would not like to wear permanently, the frowns, the squints, the scowls, the grimaces. The skin gets into a rut just as the spirits do — only these ruts are called wrinkles, and they remain long after the frown has turned into a happy smile.

One way to break these bad habits is to become aware of them. Place a strip of Scotch tape on the skin over the spot where the furrow will, or has, developed. Each time you begin to frown or pout, etc., the tape will remind you to stop. The second step is to restrict, as much as possible, the loss of moisture from the skin — the more moisture, the plumper the cell; the plumper the cell, the smoother the skin.

But first, let's examine the skin further. There are four basic types of skin: normal, dry, oily, and combination.

Chances are that, if a woman doesn't know what type of skin she has, it is normal. Normal skin is that which has neither too much oil secretion nor too little. It is firm and fairly elastic. It looks healthy and has good tone.

A dry skin tends to appear flat and flaky. It feels taut or stretched and somewhat dry to the touch. The skin appears thin and is prematurely lined with fine wrinkles. Unlike oily skin, which always looks a trifle damp and shiny, dry skin ages faster and needs more and earlier attention.

Oily skin is easily recognizable. Tiny beads of moisture (oil) cling to the surface, giving the skin a mildly greasy look. Hold a tissue to the sides of the nose, and you can actually see the oils being absorbed. The skin is somewhat more coarse and is often plagued with clogged pores and blackheads. It is less susceptible to early wrinkling and is more self-moisturizing.

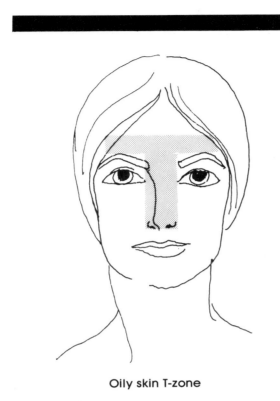

Oily skin T-zone

The only difference in these four basic types of skin is the amount of natural oil that is being secreted through the pores. Obviously, an oily skin secretes more oil than does a dry skin. It is, therefore, most important that an oily skin remain scrupulously clean to prevent oily buildup and blockage. The more cleansing, the better, to maintain open pores.

Since the secretions move outward through these pores, the channels must remain open and unrestricted. When these pores become blocked or clogged the skin develops whiteheads, blackheads, and pimples.

That is not to say that other types of skin should not be kept thoroughly clean. The same principle holds true for all types of skin. Cleanliness is next to godliness when it comes to being religious about skin care.

To convert, you must follow these nine commandments:

1. Cleanse day and night with the proper cleanser.
2. Tone the skin with the proper toner.
3. Protect the skin with a moisture cream.
4. Give the face a facial once or twice a week.
5. Keep hands away from the face.
6. Avoid excessive and habitual facial movements.
7. Maintain a balanced diet.
8. Sleep at least seven hours a night.
9. Never sunbathe or remain in the sun without first using a sun block.

A combination skin is a little bit harder to identify. This is the skin that is both dry and oily. The oily part is usually concentrated in a T-zone, that is, across the forehead and down the nose to the chin. The cheeks and under-eye areas may be flaky from dryness.

If you cannot identify your skin type, hold an eyeglass-cleaning tissue to the sides of your nose, your forehead, your cheeks. After each step, examine the tissue. Wherever the tissue turns dark from collecting and absorbing oil, you can safely assume you are oily-skinned.

DIFFERENT TYPES OF CLEANSERS AND HOW TO USE THEM

Cleansers come in a variety of forms and consistencies. The most basic of these is plain soap. The everyday soaps are most often harsh to delicate facial tissues and much too drying for all but the excessively oily skin. Soap robs the skin of its natural oils, leaving it open to chafing, scaling, and lining. Since the soap cleaning process reduces the immediate underlying well of collected oils, it is not as detrimental to oily skins as it is to the other types.

Medicated soaps are those that contain ingredients that dry the skin even more dramatically. In most cases these soaps are recommended by a dermatologist for specific reasons such as excessive oil build-up or skin eruptions. Helena Rubinstein's Bio-Clear line, however, has a medicated scrubbing bar which I particularly like.

Glycerine and super-fatted soaps, on the other hand, are gentle to the facial tissues and may be used by those who are hooked on the bar-of-soap syndrome. Neutrogena makes a fine collection of these glycerine soaps, or you might try the bar packaged under the 4711 label. Pears Soap is still a detergent-free favorite, also.

Although everyday supermarket soap is still a favorite cleansing agent for many women, only a very few should still be using it. If you are one of the addicted soap users, try instead Helena Rubinstein's Skin Life Refining Bar or Revlon's Eterna 27 Daily Cleansing Bar, which comes in two varieties: one for dry and delicate, and the other for normal skin.

Another type of cleanser is the water-soluble cream, lotion, milk, or gel. Basically, this type of cleanser is used exactly like ordinary soap, in that it is applied, mildly massaged, and then washed off with a splash of water. These cleansers are designed to be less harsh to the facial tissues, and they generally perform excellently, leaving the skin perfectly fresh, clean, and supple. Many companies produce two different types: one for dry or normal skin, and one specifically formulated for oily skin.

The Make-Up Center has three: the On Stage Floataway is a cream which may be effectively used by all skin types, while On Stage Milk Float Normal and On Stage Milk Float Oily are milky lotions which are specifically for those types of skin. Mary Quant Wash Away is a particularly pleasant foaming skin cleanser; Helena Rubinstein's Skin Life Water Activated Face Wash is efficient for oily skins; and Max Factor's Clear Cleanser with Lecithin seemed very serviceable.

Then there is the nonwater-soluble cream, sometimes called cold cream. The only difference between the two is the type of fats and emulsifiers used in the formula; one type may be dissolved in water, the other cannot. The water soluble is generally lighter in texture and is completely dissolved and washed away — with water. The nonwater-soluble is removed with cotton or — less delicate — a tissue, leaving a greasy residue. This residue must then be dissolved by the use of a skin toner.

A basic skin toner is a liquid with a variable content of water, menthol, glycerin, and alcohol. The real difference among them is the amount of alcohol in the formula — the more alcohol, the more drying the effect. This type of toner is called an astringent and should be used on oily skins. Freshener has less alcohol content and is, therefore, less drying. It is recommended for normal or dry skin.

A toner's action is to temporarily tighten the pores, recirculate the blood to the facial tissues, and temporarily remove excess natural oils. They also dissolve cold cream leftovers.

Estée Lauder makes a skin lotion which is recommended for all skin types. Her Dry Dry Skin Astringent is useful for mature and/or dry skins. I also like Clinique's Clarifying Lotion #3 for oily skin, Rubinstein's Skin Life Alcohol Free Freshener, and On Stage Freshener or Astringent.

Commercial skin toners may be replaced economically with everyday household staples. Lemon or grapefruit juice, witch hazel, and even icy water act comparatively well where there is no cold cream residue to dissolve. Fresh mint leaves steeped in water and stored in the refrigerator make an ideal toner for only pennies, too.

A toner should be applied with a cotton ball or wad (rather than with the fingertips or a tissue), avoiding the area around the eyes.

A brief moment should be spent here to explain why the use of tissues on the face is not recommended. Trace a tissue's lineage, and you will ultimately arrive at its source: wood. Soft as they may feel to the touch, tissues can be harsh to the extremely delicate skin of the face. It is, therefore, advisable to use cotton wads or balls in place of tissues or any other paper product.

Which type of cleanser is better? The prevailing belief on the one side is that the water-soluble cleanser is kinder to the skin and does a more thorough job, all in one step. There are those who also feel that each and every application of water to the face is beneficial in maintaining plump cells. They also stress that by wiping the nonwater-soluble cleanser from the skin, one tends to impact the pores, especially if careful attention to dissolving all the remaining cleanser is neglected.

Those in favor of the latter, the cold cream type of cleanser, argue that all the opposing views are sophistry. The answer, then, is to simply formulate your own opinion. Try **both** types and decide for yourself which one does the better job **for you**. Estée Lauder makes a light Whipped Cleansing Cream that is nice; their Clinique line offers Crystal Clear Cleansing Oil, which performs well, too. Pond's Cold Cream is still good. Their newer Light Whipped Cold Cream is even better.

But then I'm definitely in the water-soluble camp. However, give each type a fair trial and examine your skin closely, keeping in mind that the important thing is how well cleansed it is. In this particular case, a fair trial would mean going to the extent of using up the container. You can hardly judge after one single application — unless the product is really a loser.

The surface of the skin is not the only arena of attention. Deep-pore cleansers are a must for everyone. These grainy cleansers come in a variety of mediums: dry, powder, added to bar soap, mixed within a paste, incorporated into a cleanser. Made of almond, cornmeal, oatmeal, farina, or any other similar grain, these bits and pieces, when massaged into the skin, get down into the pores and urge the collected material forth. At the same time, these grains remove the crusty, dried tips of blackheads and blemishes, together with the outer layer of dead skin cells. When splashed away with water, the underlying layer of skin is exposed, giving the face a fresh, clean look.

The Make-Up Center's On Stage Honey & Almond Scrub smells good enough to eat and does an excellent job. Clinique's 7th Day Scrub Cream should only be used once a week, but is effective. Rubinstein's Bio-Clear Beauty Washing Grains are fine-grained and delicate. Revlon's Natural Wonder makes two serviceable bars: Super Scrub Bar for oily skin, and Gentle Scrub Bar for all other types. These grains do, however,

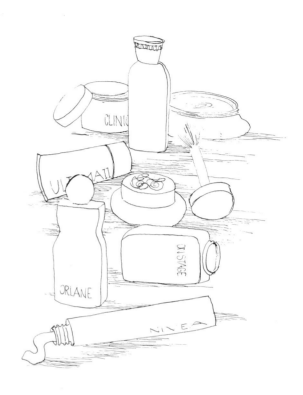

have a drying effect upon the skin and should only be used once or twice a week on normal or dry skin. Oily skin should, obviously, use them more frequently.

A facial steam bath is also very helpful for deep-pore cleansing, especially for those of us who live in cities or other highly polluted areas. Facial steamers may be purchased in a well-stocked drugstore or in most department stores.

You can achieve the same end by fabricating your own facial sauna. Boil half a panful of water. Remove the pan from the heat and, protecting your legs with towels, place the pan on your lap. With your hair pinned back, cover your head and the pan on your lap with a large bath towel. The steam that collects under this barrier will open your pores, allowing the collected matter to be more easily secreted or removed. Glemby's Herbal Concentrate adds a delicious essense or you might like to create your own, by adding a few herbs to the water as you boil it. Two or three cloves and a dash of nutmeg do nothing for your skin, but the fragrance will heighten your spirits. And anything that makes us feel better makes us look better!

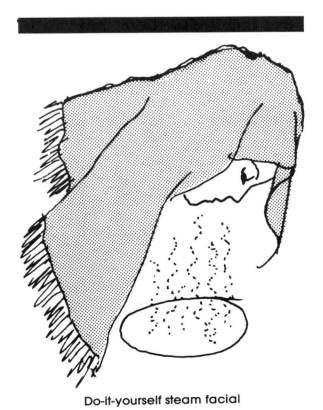

Do-it-yourself steam facial

FACIAL MASKS

The use of a mask (masque) is another boon to keeping the skin fresh and clean. A facial mask helps to "vacuum" the pores. There are several types of masks, from gels to packs, liquids to creams. In essense, they all do the same thing; the only difference is the degree to which they function. The basic role of a mask is performed while the mixture dries on the face. As the moisture in the mask evaporates, the mask dries and hardens. The pores are squeezed slightly, and the natural oils or impacted matter is urged outward. This action also stimulates the flow of blood to the skin, and the blood, in turn, carries its supply of oxygen. The mask forms a barrier and the moisture in the cells accumulates, plumping up the skin. As the skin plumps up, the pores become smaller. The outer layer of dead cells is removed by the mask, and the pores are dramatically "tightened."

Unfortunately, this tightening action is very short-lived. As soon as the collected moisture oxidizes, the skin returns to its original state. **There is nothing that can be done to shrink pores permanently.** The urgent need is to prevent them from becoming more distended and engorged, thereby enlarging them.

Masks are designed for all types of skin, from dry to oily. The Make-Up Center's cleansing and firming masque is On Stage Mud Pie with Pectin. While the mask is

Their Clinique line has one called Beauty Emergency Mask, which may be used every day on oily skins. Helena Rubinstein has a competent Fresh Cover Clay Cleanser and their Skin Life line has an effective Clarifying Mineral Mask for oily skins.

Another type of mask is the nutritional variety. These are the masks that do not harden on the skin and do not perform any tightening action. Their purpose is to "feed" the skin. On Stage Wheat Germ & Kelp Nourisher is actually a food that may be eaten, but its purpose is to nourish the skin with the proteins and minerals available in its ingredients. On Stage also makes a tranquilizing mask, Camomile & Zinc Calmer. Its purpose is to do for the skin what a sedative does for the psyche. A boon to troubled, sensitive, or irritated skin, it is a lovely soother for normal skin as well.

The directions for the use of any mask should be followed carefully. Care must also be taken with certain peel-off masks to insure that the hair of the brows and the hairline is not pulled away with the film. No drying mask should **ever** be applied to the area around the eyes. This is one of the spots on the face that never self-replenishes its moisture content. For that reason it is the first area to form the fine "laugh lines" that later become full-fledged wrinkles. It is, therefore, most important that **everybody** apply a moisture cream to this sensitive area. Everybody includes teenagers and men, too!

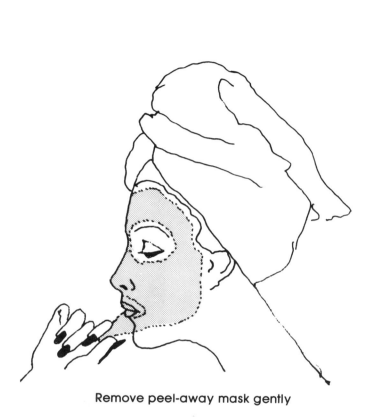

Remove peel-away mask gently

performing all the actions described above, it is also nourishing the skin with the citrus vitamins plus the rare vitamin P found in the pulp (the pectin) of the orange. Estée Lauder has a lovely Almond Clay Pack.

MOISTURIZERS

To understand why this is so important, you must first understand the role of a moisture cream. A good moisture cream attracts and holds water in the cells, while preventing the loss of moisture through normal oxidation. As reviewed before, the more plump the skin cells, the more puffed out the skin. The more puffed out the skin, the smoother it looks and the shallower the existing lines appear.

Picture a balloon. Inflated with air, its surface is taut, creaseless, and smooth. Empty, its surface is flabby, wrinkled. The moisture in the skin is relative to the air in the balloon.

In keeping with this principle, a veil of moisture cream should be applied day and night to most skins. For this reason, most companies produce more than one type of cream, in more than one consistency.

A daytime moisturizer is generally light, nongreasy, and quickly absorbed. It forms a protective layer between the skin and make-up, pollution, windburn, etc.

The Make-Up Center produces two fine moisturizers for use under make-up. On Stage Underbase is designed for young or normal skins; On Stage Enriched Moisture is a cream for dry or mature skins. I also like Estée Lauder's Enriched Under Make-Up Creme and Max Factor's Geminesse, Living Proof Hydracel Moisturizer. The Mary Quant Skin Saver is called a night moisturizer, but I find it good for under make-up protection for dry skin, as well.

A nighttime moisturizer does not have to be much thicker, nor does it have to be greasy to be effective. It is, however, usually somewhat thicker than a daytime cream but should still maintain good penetrating qualities. Jacqueline Cochran's Flowing Velvet has long been a favorite. Charles of the Ritz's Revenescence Moist Environment Night Treatment is very functional, as is Noxzema's Raintree Moisture Concentrate.

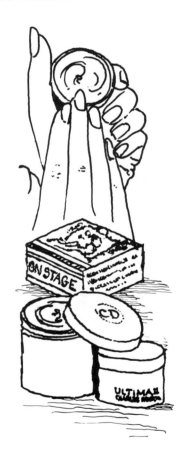

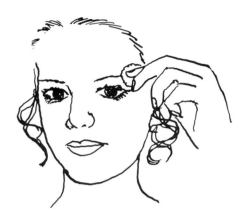

I also like Revlon's Dry Skin Relief Moisture Lotion for normal and combination skins and their Formula 2, Programs A and B. My favorite, of course, is the On Stage Renewal ; it's jam-packed with every conceivable goodie for the restoration of the skin. The On Stage Super Nourish is the normal, combination, or young skin nighttime moisturizer. I say "nighttime" because that was its original concept. I know several women, however, who use nighttime moisturizers for daytime under their make-up. There are no rules when it comes to the adaptation of products, and you should not feel uncertain or afraid to experiment.

Frankly, if I could not afford a moisture cream, per se, I would feel some reassurance that I was doing **something** to retard wrinkling by merely applying plain old Vaseline! Does that mean that plain Vaseline is as good as the higher priced moisture creams? Of course not. In most cases, it

definitely is not — but it **is** as good as some of the products that are currently on the market! That is why it is so urgent that you sample-test and research for yourself rather than simply accept all claims.

What am I saying here? Basically, it boils down to this. Now that the law requires that cosmetic ingredients be listed, it makes it easy for you to compare products. You don't have to be in the dark any longer, relying wholly upon the company's integrity. See for yourself. There is a book available that is very helpful. **A Consumer's Dictionary of Cosmetic Ingredients** is compiled by Ruth Winter and published by Crown Publishers. You can look up just about every cosmetic ingredient listed on your cosmetic package and find out just exactly what's what. Find out what these chemicals do, and you have the important data on that particular product.

Cosmetic products are not as complicated as they may seem to the uninitiated. I sometimes think that the confusion is 90 percent of the magnitude of the products available. Truth to tell, there are not that many different cosmetic companies. The confusion lies in the fact that the large cosmetic companies — which, in turn, are part of even larger conglomerates — issue several different lines of cosmetics. Revlon has Natural Wonder, Revlon, Ultima, and Charlie. Helena Rubinstein has Skin Life, Skin Dew, Bio-Clear, Existence, Ultra Feminine; Estée Lauder has Estée Lauder and Clinique, Max Factor has Geminesse, etc., etc., etc. To name them all would be boring.

What's the purpose? Well, in some cases, the lines are priced differently so as to reach the broadest spectrum of the market. Sometimes the lines are priced differently **and** geared to different age brackets. Sometimes it's as simple as one line having heavy fragrance and one having none at all. There are all sorts of reasons. What it signifies is a lot of confusion and the necessity to take a little time and effort before purchasing. You wouldn't buy just any old car, or meat, or medication. Take the same precautions with make-up.

The important factor in judging a moisture cream is to analyze its effectiveness by examining the skin an hour or so after its application. Has the cream been completely absorbed? Does the skin feel taut and stretched, or soft and supple? Does it feel dry to the touch? Does the face have a greasy, slick feel?

What do you look for? A good moisture cream penetrates fairly rapidly and leaves the skin feeling soft and moist for hours. The old-fashioned notion that a woman must go to bed with a thick layer of cream on her face is just that — old-fashioned.

A newer trend, supported by many health fadists, is the belief that **no** moisture cream at all should be applied at night, thereby allowing the skin to "breathe." In truth, the skin's ability to "breathe" has little or nothing to do with a moisture cream **unless**, of course, the cream in question is so dense it impacts the pores. In that case, the use of a moisture cream is obviously detrimental rather than beneficial.

Another fallacy is the belief that people with oily skin should never use a moisture cream. It is quite true that people with oily skin do not need **as much** moisture fed back into the skin as do normal- or dry-skinned people. They have abundant natural oils, and their skin remains plump and youthful-looking much longer. Oily skin **does**, however, need supportive moisture in those areas that do not produce their own supply — under the eyes, on the cheeks, and on the neck.

Moisture creams are made of a variety of ingredients. The basic ingredient in a good cream is a substance which holds or attracts water. These substances are called **natural moisturizing factors**. There are creams made with estrogen or collagen, avocado oil and mink oil, vitamins A, D, E — plus a myriad other nourishing and beneficial ingredients. One should experiment widely **and only then** make an educated selection. Choose the cream that does the most for your own specific requirements and, in most cases, completely ignore and disregard the exaggerated claims of advertising copy.

Cream should be applied sparingly. The assumption that if a little does such good, a lot will do much more is erroneous. Using your index finger, dot the nose, the chin, the cheeks with the cream. Using the fingertips, gently blend the dots of cream all over the face and neck, paying particular attention to the area under and around the eyes.

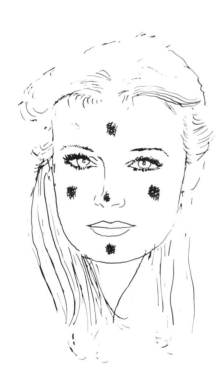

Apply moisture cream in dots

Remember your collagen fibers! Don't rub and press, causing the skin under your fingers to shift grotesquely. Instead, blend lightly so that you are smoothing the cream on, rather than rubbing it in. Never pull the face downward (let gravity work its own misery). Don't be constantly on guard or compulsive about it, however. Just try to get into the habit of lateral and/or upward motions.

What about special eye creams? There are those who feel that a finer textured cream should be applied to the eye area or that this sensitive area requires different ingredients than those available in the normal moisturizer. I do not agree with this theory, preferring to hold the opinion that, if it's a good moisturizer, it can be used all over the face and give the same benefits. There are, however, several eye creams on the market, and you should test them in order to formulate your own opinion. Skin Life has an Eye Wrinkle Stick that has the advantage of being handy to use.

I would like to remark about the very obvious lack of skin care products within the less expensive lines. These are the lines that are so handily blister-packed and hung on racks just about everywhere you shop. Although these lines (Maybelline, Revlon, Max Factor, Coty, Love, etc., etc.) are not extensive in their color lines compared to the cosmetics available behind the counter, I find the lack of any cleansers, creams, or treatments a more serious omission — one that I hope will soon be remedied. It's no wonder we Americans are so Johnny-come-lately in our attention to skin care. It's been limited to those who could afford it! (Except, of course, for those of you who already knew about On Stage!

While I'm on the subject I would also like to voice my opinion about those blister-packed cosmetics. I think the marketing is swell, but I also think the lack of an open sample for testing creates a lot of money wasted on items that the purchaser did not discover were unsuitable until **after** she got them home. It is so very important that you sample a product to see if the color is correct, the texture suitable, the smell pleasant, and the coverage acceptable **before** you actually buy it. It just makes me angry. It's like being forced into either buying a more expensive, counter-available product or buying a pig in a poke! That's what it really is, since you never know exactly what you're buying until after you have!

To return to more pleasant things, there is another way to speed you on the way to healthy skin, not an alternative but a supplement — the facial salon.

Modern techniques and machinery are a definite plus in the quest for good skin. At first glance the machinery of the esthetician seems strange and very much like something from a Boris Karloff laboratory. Once you get to know the functions of the equipment, however, you will see how basic are their operations. The following is a rundown on what you can expect on a visit to a facial salon.

GETTING A FACIAL

A typical treatment begins with the removal of make-up and soil from the skin. This is usually accomplished with cotton wads and a mild cleanser. Then the esthetician examines the skin. There are two methods. One is the use of a Wood lamp. This is a black light that transforms the skin color to a ghostly purple shade. The trained eye can see the different shadings of spotted white, brown, and orange that reveal what lies within the skin. Another method for analysis is the magnified, lighted glass. Sometimes the esthetician may use both tools. In any event and with any method, skin analysis is vital in determining what treatment to employ. The esthetician must determine if the pores are enlarged, if blackheads exist, if any blemishes are apparent or lying just below the surface, and what **type** of skin lies under her hand. Is it dehydrated? Are there wrinkles? What is the condition of the capillaries? Does excess sebum exist? What is the condition of the elasticity of the tissues? Is there any discoloration, excess hair, pressure sensitivity? These are all important, because the skin type determines the treatment.

The first of the mechanical operations is the cleansing of the skin, beyond what has already been done manually. A cleansing machine normally has a wand with an assortment of goat's-hair brushes and a pumice-stone attachment. These are all used to slough off the dead skin cells, the encrusted pore caps, and any soil that remained after the manual cleansing.

Afterward, the vaporizer is initiated. A gentle, fine mist of warm, ionized water

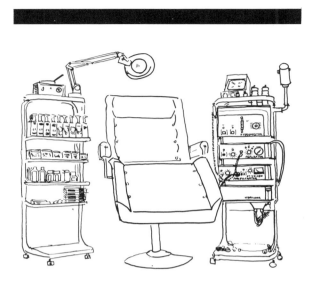

One type of professional facial machinery

vapor is directed toward the face, producing a four-fold action: it relaxes the tissues; it urges the pores to open; it stimulates blood circulation; and it moisturizes on a temporary basis. The vapor treatment lasts ten to fifteen minutes. Now that the pores are opened, a mild abrasive is applied to deep-clean the pores. This is usually a grainy cleanser.

Then a treatment called **desincrustation** may follow. Desincrustation is the removal of sebum, the oily mass secreted by the sebaceous glands, via the employment of stabilized galvanic current. Galvanic current is the medium through which an experienced esthetician can penetrate the skin's

natural barrier. This penetration is called **iontophoresis**. Through iontophoresis, it is possible to drive the active principles of products, in the shape of ions, past the skin's barrier and into the inner layer of the subcutaneous tissue. For the desincrustation treatment, a special liquid that dissolves sebum is driven into the skin.

The client holds, or rests upon, one pole while the esthetician works with the opposing pole. The end of the instrument is covered with a cotton wad which has been saturated with the specially designed liquid. The wad is replaced several times during the treatment.

A gentle pinching or kneading of the skin can follow to aid in the release of oil from the pores and to empty the sebaceous glands. Then the skin can be vacuumed. Small glass tubes (**ventouse**) are applied to the face, to remove the now liquefied sebum or other trapped soil, loosened blackheads, pollution, etc. If there are pimples present, the esthetician may place the suction directly over the infected area for spot vacuuming — or she may employ yet another machine.

This machine utilizes high frequency to produce thermal current. Ultraviolet rays of high-frequency current sterilize the skin's eruptions. A process called **sparking** may individually treat each blemish. A small current of electricity is transmitted to the pimple, creating a tiny spark. This spark helps to dry and heal the active blemish while also having a germicidal action.

Now that the skin has been thoroughly deep-cleaned, a good facial continues with the application of a mask. As mentioned before, there are several types of masks, hardening and nonhardening. A good esthetician will not give you the same treatment each time you visit. If she **does,** you are not getting the full benefit of all the products on the market and the extensive variety of the machines. Among the other types of masks may be those that are designed for nourishment only. These masks may not harden. They are applied and allowed to stand for ten to twenty minutes, giving the tissues time to absorb the nutrients. Sometimes the esthetician will apply this thick, gruel-type mask over cheesecloth to facilitate removal.

Or rather than use a nutritional mask, the esthetician may elect to help restore the skin by employing galvanic current and a penetrating solution. These solutions tone the tissues, renew cellular action, rejuvenate, prevent allergic reactions, act on acne skins, help heal broken capillaries, promote rehydration, and as already mentioned, liquefy sebum. The galvanic current also increases circulation, regulates muscle tone, improves metabolism, and increases the flow of blood and lymphatic circulation.

Whenever these machines (either the galvanic or the high-frequency current) are employed, they must be operated by a trained, experienced esthetician. Make sure yours is qualified!

How do you know? Read reputable publications, **Harper's Bazaar, Vogue,** **Cosmopolitan, Mademoiselle.** Sophisticated magazines such as these have beauty departments that do excellent reporting on what's available. Usually they actually test to know that what they're saying is true, so you can feel safe in taking their advice. Ask your doctor or call a dermatologist to see if either can recommend a facial salon. Listen to what people say, but don't be influenced without checking up. The machinery used in facial salons can be dangerous. Too much current can produce a burn (and a scar) and can also disturb the electrical impulses of the body. People who wear pacemakers, have bad hearts, poor circulation, etc., should, of course, not submit to any galvanic current processes. A reputable firm should ask you your health condition before performing any of these services.

Normally, the step that follows the mask is the massage. There are several ways to give this massage: by hand, by vibrating machine, or by hand via high frequency.

The massage by hand is, of course, the manipulation of the skin by the esthetician's fingertips, pure, simple, and delicious! The vibrating machine technique is delightful, too, and it is done by placing a machine on top of the hand. The vibrations are then transmitted through the hand onto the client's skin. The high-frequency method is a variation of this, but milder and less vigorous. The client holds a special electrode that is connected to the high-frequency machine. The touch of the esthetician then becomes the source of vibration. A practiced, professional operator can make this part of the facial the highlight of your day!

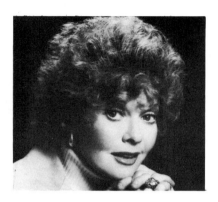

I use masks of every kind, including homemade ones I make myself. If I'm using an avocado in a recipe, whatever's left over after scooping out the shell goes on my face, and if there's enough, on my hands too. Or, if a banana is handy and I'm not eating it (I love them), it can go on my face too. I also make up a mask out of 100 percent wheat germ flour, vitamin E oil, and a little milk or cream or just water if I have nothing else. I put on a thin coating and let it dry. Then I rinse it off with cold water alternating with lukewarm water and finish off with a healthy amount of some kind of rich oil.

JANIS PAIGE

The purpose of the massage is to invigorate the muscles, stimulate the blood circulation, and moisturize. A good nonvanishing cream should be applied that is worked into the skin through the warmth of gentle friction caused by the manipulation. Some machinery comes equipped with a facial iron. The iron is heated hot; its surface is coated with the cream; and then the hot iron is quickly passed over the face, never theoretically, being left in one spot long enough to burn. This "irons out" the wrinkles. I don't believe it to that extent, but it **does** help the moisturizer to penetrate, and it feels like heaven!

To be perfectly truthful, all the claims made by the manufacturers of these facial machines should be examined closely before you completely accept them. The cleansing equipment is definitely a valid and proven theory, and the sterilization via high frequency makes perfect sense and has also been tested and proven. The galvanic-current operation has **not,** to my knowledge, been adequately studied and proven. It **sounds** like it should work, but I'm not a chemist or a scientist. I would like to see some actual before-and-afters before I put **all** my faith in its effects!

After the massage, a refreshing spray of skin toner to close the pores and, alas, it's over. (You can tell that I'm a facial freak. Once you feel how wonderful they are, you will be, too!)

But don't get upset if the facial you pay for is not exactly like the one I've described. Remember, estheticians are people, and variety is what makes horse races crumble — or something like that. I **would** recommend, however, that you go to a salon that has some type of machinery; you really do get more of a facial from them.

Many facial salons offer a make-up session after the skin care treatment has been completed. Do not hesitate to enjoy (and maybe learn from) this service. Applying make-up directly after a facial is not detrimental to the skin. There is no harmful effect, and, as a matter of fact, high-quality make-up further protects the skin!

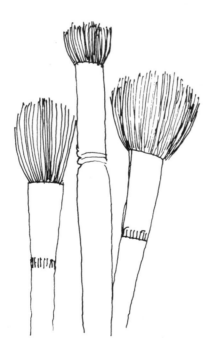

BLEMISH PROBLEMS

Before this chapter closes, a word should be said about acne.

A healthy skin is one which has open, constantly active pores. The amount of material flowing through these pores depends upon the individual. As long as the pores are clear, however, no pustules or wens will develop. When the passageways are plugged, a **comedo** (a pimple) or blackhead forms. The important thing, therefore, is to keep the skin clean without robbing it of all its natural moisture.

Acne is a condition of severe pore blockage. It is brought about by a change in the body, by puberty, by the release of sex hormones, and by overactive glands. Mild acne can spontaneously clear up without any damage to the skin. Severe cases, however, involve repeated infection and irritation. This type of acne may last well into the twenties and usually causes irreversible scarring. Unfortunately, there is no cure-all. Vitamin A, tetracycline, drugstore lotions, creams, and elixirs may help some lucky few but only irritate others further.

Acne cannot be cured because, as of yet, it is somewhat of a medical mystery. The mystery is why do the pores or ducts, which are the normal route for the lubricant, become clogged?

Dr. Alan Shalita, the head of dermatology at State University of New York's Downstate Medical Center, has a theory that there are certain people who react to something in the skin's natural oils or some action of bacteria on oil or both. Their follicle cells become hard and gluey, thereby refusing to slough off the skin. This causes a blockage which, in turn, causes blackheads.

Until science discovers its answers, we can only try to "control" acne. The way to do that is to:

1. Wash the skin three and four times a day. Scrubbing is unnecessary and may cause more irritation.
2. Resist the temptation to squeeze with the fingertips. There are comedo extractors that are safer to use. Ask your doctor.
3. Shampoo the hair every day. If possible, wear the hair away from the face. If not, make sure it is always clean.
4. Eat a well-balanced diet. If certain foods create a flare-up, stop eating them! The long-standing beliefs that chocolate, cola drinks, masturbation, lack of sex, or pent-up feelings developed into acne are untrue.
5. Get out into the sun — but don't burn. The sun has a natural drying effect.
6. Do not wear greasy, heavy make-up to conceal the condition. It works in reverse. Light, water-based foundations can more deceptively hide mild blemishes.
7. Do not lean your face on your hands. No, it's not altogether because of the bacteria transfer; the pressure itself can cause skin problems.

For a medicated cleanser, Westwood Pharmaceuticals produces Fostex Liquid Medicated Skin Cleanser, which I think performs well. Neutrogena Acne Cleansing Soap is a mild, unmedicated bar that's good, too. Contrary to popular belief, very strong soaps or detergents are actually bad for the acne-prone skin and definitely cause acne flare-ups. Be gentle when you wash your face, and do not scrub with a barkcloth (Tawashi) or rough washcloth.

Basically, the three definite **musts** when it comes to acne-prone skin are:

1. The excess oil must be dissolved.
2. The dead skin cells must be sloughed off.
3. The healing process must be accelerated.

Now that the federal government has ruled that cosmetic companies must list the ingredients of the cosmetic on the package, it is simple to select products that contain particular chemicals that will be effective.

Look for alcohol, which dries up excess oils and also acts as a disinfectant. Resorcinol and salicylic acid are good peeling agents that remove the outer layer of dead skin cells that clog pores. Sulfur helps to speed up the healing process, as does aloe vera and tocopherols (vitamin E) — just to name a few. Helena Rubinstein's Bio-Clear Medicated Stick and Clearasil Acne Pimple Stick Medication cover as well as help to dry up superficial blemishes.

As for the scarring caused by acne, the only really effective remedy for deep pockets, or anything more than can be concealed with cosmetics, is the dermatologist and the plastic surgeon. There are peeling and sanding and grafting procedures that the doctor can describe in great detail.

If you have broken capillaries, they are in the dermatologist's domain, too. Do not let anyone else treat them. For those of you who do have them and wonder how they got there, there are three possible ways. Or a combination of all three is highly possible: an acute change of temperature (for instance, coming from a warm house into frigid, blustering winds); a trauma; by aggressive squeezing of pimples or blackheads.

A dermatologist can easily rid you of these red, threadlike lines by inserting a high-frequency needle into the capillary which dries the blood and stops the flow. You should, of course, consult a doctor to make sure that these broken capillaries are not a medical problem, and you should always have a professional treat them.

There are two other areas of skin problems that should be discussed here briefly. Those of you who are confronted with these problems should see a dermatologist for more in-depth information and advice.

One is the condition generally termed a "ruddy complexion." This is the skin that always seems rosy-red or flushed. This type of condition is called **rosacea.** It defines the inflamed skin that is generally caused by several different factors. Top on the list is stress. Second is spicy foods, alcohol, and coffee — all of which can do an inflammation job on their own but added to frustration create a powerful weapon. The treatment is a prescription from your doctor or dermatologist for antibiotics. Some prescribe a lotion to be applied to the skin, and others prefer induction via the mouth; sometimes

both methods are recommended. Discuss this fully, as all your questions, with a qualified source.

The other problem is really no problem at all; it just seems like one. These are the tiny red dots or spots you may notice on your skin. These resemble tiny insect bites or dark red birthmarks. They are called **cherry angiomas** and are harmless collections of capillaries that sit on top of the skin. They suddenly appear and may or may not disappear. About 85 percent of the population over thirty years of age gets them, and they turn up anywhere. A doctor can remove them very easily, if desired, with an electric needle or with liquid nitrogen. If, however, you have an angioma that changes in appearance you should see your doctor about it as soon as possible.

There is another thing you can do to retard the aging process and to maintain healthy, clear skin — protect the skin from the harmful rays of the sun. We are all consumed with the idea that we are more beautiful and more healthy looking with a glorious tan. The aesthetics of the question are moot; the health angle is quite another thing. The sun can cause skin cancer. It's as simple as that. The sun also can make the skin look like the desert in the middle of July. It can make the skin look like unpolished leather and carve lines into the face that resemble the craters on the moon!

The answer is to be **extraordinarily** careful about protecting your skin when you are out in the sun, whether you are sun bathing, walking to work, or out on a picnic. There are special suntan lotions with ingredients that not only moisturize the skin but

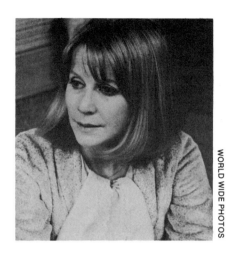

WORLD WIDE PHOTOS

I generally cleanse with Nivea and I moisturize my face with Lancome's Lancomia Creme. My favorite beauties when I was a kid were Vivien Leigh and Anna Magnani; the one feature I would have loved to have had was big brown eyes. On my own eyes I use a brown eye contour color, a tiny bit of white cream eyeshadow on the lid, eyeliner, and **three** coats of black mascara. I use a foundation shade to lighten my complexion, and sometimes I add powder. When I wear lipstick or lipgloss, it's always in a pale color.

JULIE HARRIS

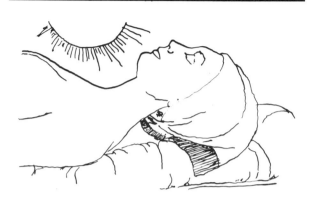

Protect your skin with a good sun-blocking agent

also block out the harmful rays. On Stage Underbase is just such a cream. You can also go to your druggist, who can offer PABA (para-aminobenzoic acid), which you can apply to serve the same purpose.

Tan slowly; do not burn your skin. And moisturize, moisturize, moisturize! When you come in from outdoors or even as you continue whatever activity keeps you in the sun, smooth on an adequate film of cream all over your exposed body. Be sure to re-place this sun-block after bathing.

A PROGRAM FOR HEALTHY SKIN

Your skin is only as good as its care and preservation. Regardless of how good it is — or becomes — proper care must be taken to maintain it. Every day and every week, regimens **must** be sustained!

To review what that program should be:

NORMAL OR DRY SKIN

EVERY DAY

Morning:
1. CLEANSE.

2. TONE.

3. MOISTURIZE.

Bedtime:
4. CLEANSE.

5. TONE.

6. MOISTURIZE.

EVERY WEEK

Give yourself an at-home facial.
1. CLEANSE.

2. USE FACIAL SAUNA.

3. USE DEEP PORE CLEANSING GRAINS.

4. APPLY A MASK.

5. MOISTURIZE

OILY SKIN

EVERY DAY

Morning:
1. CLEANSE.

2. TONE.

3. MOISTURIZE.

Bedtime:
4. CLEANSE.

5. TONE.

6. MOISTURIZE.

EVERY WEEK

Give yourself at least two facials.
1. CLEANSE.

2. USE FACIAL SAUNA.

3. USE DEEP PORE CLEANSING GRAINS.

4. APPLY A SELF-DRYING MASK.

5. APPLY A SOOTHING MASK.

6. MOISTURIZE.

COMBINATION SKIN: FOLLOW THE REGIMEN FOR NORMAL SKIN.

CARING FOR YOUR SKIN

Following these simple instructions, you should arrive at clear, smooth skin. But don't expect miracles. The treatment takes time and effort. And don't be discouraged if you see more and more pimples after a treatment. In most cases, this disturbance is caused by the underlying irritations that the facials have brought up to the surface to be dispelled. They will soon disappear altogether if you simply maintain the program and have patience.

Please don't be too quick to assume that the new pimples are a reaction to the products themselves, either. Of course it is possible that you are allergic to one or more of the ingredients in a product, in which case you should discontinue its use. But don't jump to conclusions. If you are normally sensitive, you are probably already aware that you break out in allergic reaction. You will, of course, examine the ingredients within a product before its purchase.

Those of you who are not normally sensitized should not immediately assume that it's the product that is at fault — that is, without first objectively examining your own conduct. Are those pimples really the result of applying the product? Or is it those french fries, that pepperoni pizza, the one or two nights you were too tired to remove your make-up, the fact that you haven't exactly followed a good health program because you hate vegetables and don't believe all that stuff about a proper diet to begin with? How about that fight with your boyfriend or the anxiety because of the new responsibilities laid upon you at work or menstruation or the fact that your in-laws are coming to visit?

It is virtually impossible to have a totally hypoallergenic product. Some people are even sensitive to water! Most reputable cosmetic companies cautiously omit all known irritants from their product manufacture but, truthfully, there can still be allergic reactions.

In most cases this reaction is to the fragrance included in the product to mask or cover any disagreeable chemical odors. Fragrance sensitivity far exceeds any other type of reaction. Haven't you ever experienced a slight headache or nausea after being confined in an elevator or other restricted area with someone whose scent disturbed you? For this reason, many companies are now producing fragrance-free cosmetics. Revlon is producing such a line. Clinique is, perhaps, the forerunner.

A good way to test the product for sensitivity reaction is to apply a little to the inside of your wrist, cover with a Band-Aid, and see what happens in a couple of hours. If your skin under the Band-Aid breaks out into a rash you have definite proof that there is something in the product to which you are sensitive.

But, for goodness sakes, don't dump all your skin problems in the "I'm allergic" basket. It's the lazy way out, and it may not be true at all!

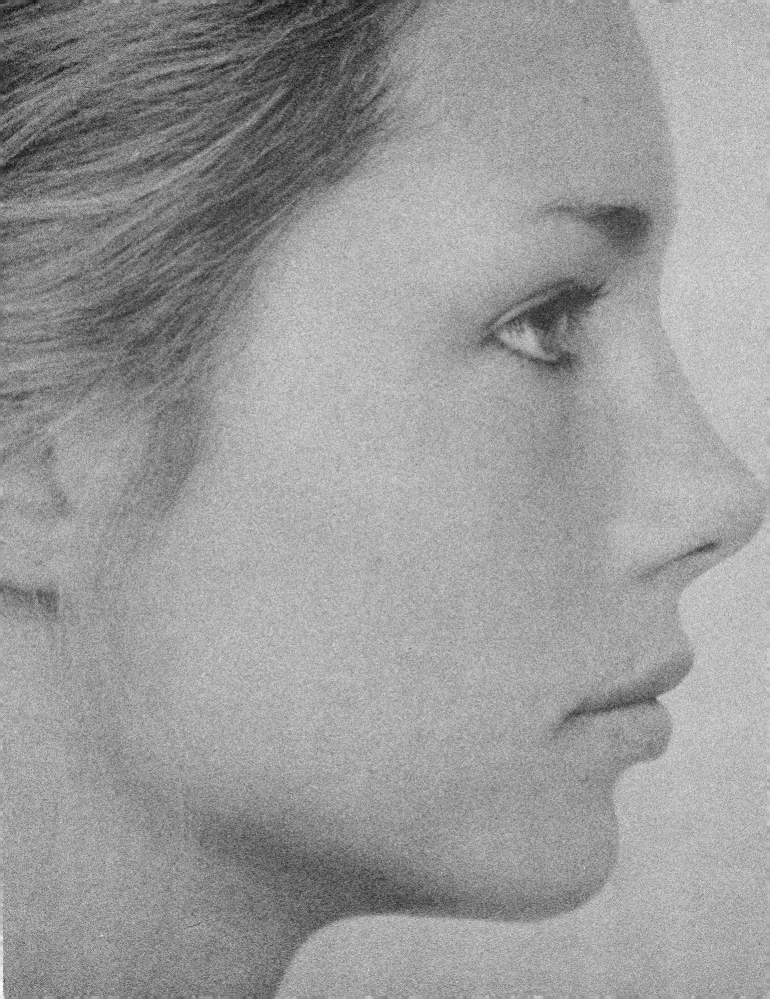

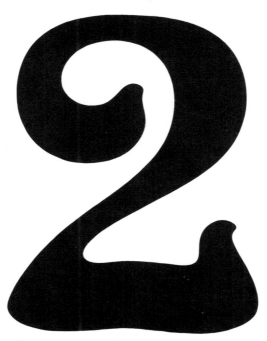

HOW TO DO YOUR OWN COMPLETE STEP-BY-STEP MAKE-OVER

HOW TO HIDE CIRCLES UNDER THE EYES

One of the first steps in the totally acceptable and widely practiced deception of making up is to conceal the circles under the eyes. In order to do this effectively, you must first become aware of the principle of **chiaroscuro**: the play of light and dark.

You are probably already consciously or subconsciously aware of the following very simple optical illusion. When you wear a black dress, you look much thinner than when you wear a white dress, right? In the diagram below, the black rectangle looks much smaller than the white rectangle, isn't that true?

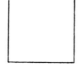

The answer is simple. Light or bright colors make an object or an area seem larger and closer to the observing eye. Dark and dull colors make the same area appear smaller and farther away. Well, this principle is applied time and time again in the art of applying make-up professionally. It is called highlighting and contouring.

Almost all of us have circles under our eyes. It has nothing to do with dissipation or "high living." Nor has it anything whatsoever to do with growing old, which is one redeeming factor. It is an inherited trait, and there is little one can do about it except treat it cosmetically. Even a twelve-year-old can look drawn and peaked because of these circles! The answer, then, is obvious. Hide them!

To define these circles: they are usually a dull, bluish or gray color and are shades darker than the surrounding skin. What is needed is to lighten, or "highlight" these discolored areas.

There are several products on the market that have been designed especially for this purpose. Some are liquid; others are creams; still others are gels, pastes, or cream pastes. By and large, the mode of application is identical; the only difference is the degree to which they are effective. You must experiment with all types, because the effectiveness of **any** product is directly related to your ability to use it.

Max Factor's Erase comes in a tube and several different shades. Cover Girl has a nice Undereye Cover Stick, and so does Love, the Under Eye Cover, which comes in a tube. More expensive but just as nice is Clinique's Concealing Stick, also in a tube. My favorite, my unbiased favorite, is the On Stage Touch, because it provides a sheer veil of concealment that stays put and does not form greasy lines.

The most popular type of concealer is the cream variety. It remains in place without fading, shifting or creasing if applied correctly. Because it is applied under the foundation, this type of concealer is off-white in color. The foundation, which is blended over the concealer, hides this shade difference. This same concealer therefore may be worn by women of all complexion tones.

If you prefer to use a concealer that is designed to be used **over** the foundation, make sure that the shade is exact, so that no line of demarcation is shown around the area of its application.

In either case, the mode of application is fairly precise. The circle or discoloration, **and it alone**, should be covered by the concealer. That is to say, do not extend the application upward into the lash root or sideways to the corner of the eye **unless** the discoloration actually lies there.

With a Q-Tip or a piece of cotton wrapped around an orange stick dab a small amount of the concealer onto the area. Remember that this area is extremely fragile. Lines and wrinkles, if they're not already there, will form soon enough without you promoting them by dragging and pulling the skin. Dot the concealer on first one eye and then the other, leaving small spaces in between each little dot. Now, reverse the Q-Tip so that the clean end is exposed. Proceed to gently pat and blend the concealer until a thin, even film has been applied.

It is very important that you learn to apply just the right thickness of the particular product you have selected. Too much cream or paste will look greasy and made-up, forming disagreeable lines of collected cream the first time the skin is shifted into a smile. Too much liquid and

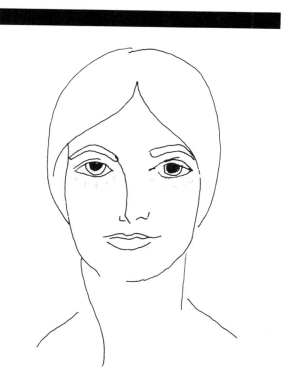

Dots of concealer

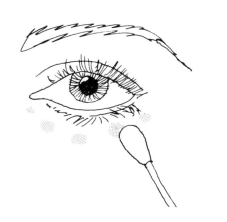

Apply with Q-tip

your finished product will resemble an owl. The proper coverage leaves the once-discolored area a shade or two lighter than the surrounding skin.

Minor facial blemishes, birthmarks, and even fine lines may also be concealed with the same careful attention. In the case of lines, however, a fine brush, like a #00, should be employed in place of the rather blunt Q-Tip. Since the line is recessed into the skin, the line itself is in shadow. What you want to do is artificially bring more light to that area. Trace each line, being careful you do not extend the application of the concealer to any of the surrounding skin. The fine hairs of the brush should lightly touch only the crease itself. Do not put on a heavy layer. Now, using a Q-Tip, pat each line until the edges have been feathered and the concealer has been blended evenly.

HOW TO APPLY THE FOUNDATION

You are now ready to prepare the background. And that is precisely how you should regard a foundation (or base as it is sometimes called). Foundation provides the backdrop for all your subtle and/or colorful artistry.

The sole purpose of a foundation is to give the face one even color tone. In selecting the proper shade, it is essential that you match, as closely as possible, the shade of the complexion.

In **certain** cases, however, this is inadvisable. Sometimes the complexion is too ruddy, too sallow, or, perhaps, much too uneven to try to camouflage. In these cases the use of a corrective pigmentation regulator is needed under the foundation. These regulators are called **toners** and should not be confused with the skin toners which were discussed previously. (You will meet with more than one ambivalence as you become more and more familiar with cosmetic jargon.)

These toners or regulators usually come in liquid or cream form and in four basic colors: green, red, violet, and white. Some of these toners have moisturizing qualities, in which case the application of the moisture cream before the application of the under-eye concealer may be omitted.

In order to understand how toners work, we must first review the color wheel and its cycle. Perhaps you remember making one of these in grammar school. There are three **primary colors**: red, yellow, and blue. The colors directly opposite these primary colors on the color wheel are called **complementary colors**. They are green, violet, and orange. These colors work to intensify each other when they are placed side by side or to minimize or subdue each other when they are placed one on top of the other.

For a ruddy complexion, therefore, the application of a green toner reduces the amount of redness in the skin. A sallow or yellow complexion loses its jaundiced undertones with a violet toner. The blotchy dark and light complexion is aided by the white toner, and the grayish, drab undertones in some black skins are minimized by the red toner.

This toner is applied just as if it were the moisture cream (if it is of that type) or directly over the moisture cream. Either one goes **under** the foundation. It should be applied sparingly so that too thick a cover is not applied to the skin but, instead, merely a translucent coating. Pay particular attention to the hairline and the creases of the nose and chin. The moisturized variety may be smoothed on with the fingertips; the other should be applied with a dry foam sponge. The choice of a foundation shade is then selected to match the corrected facial color tone, generally a pure beige.

All other complexions should be matched so that a dot of foundation placed on the cheek is fairly invisible from a pace away from the mirror. The practice of trying to match a complexion shade by testing a foundation on the wrist or hand is totally and completely misguided. The color tones of the skin in both areas are, in most cases, completely different than that of the face. It is also impossible to try to match your complexion by looking at a color swatch on a sample card. First of all, the ink used in representing the shade of foundation can never be exact. Second, the shade will look entirely different when it is applied to the skin rather than to a clear, white pasteboard.

Judging the proper shade of foundation for a white skin is fairly simple if you have a good eye. The selection for a black skin is not that simple, unfortunately. First of all, the variations of black skin have a ratio of about three to one in comparison with white skin. You look at a white skin and can immediately see the undertones: tinges of yellow, pink, red, even blue. On a black skin, these undertones are not always so easily identifiable.

Through practice, of course, the eye can be trained to see one's underlying tones and thereby help in the proper selection of a foundation. Until such time, however, a careful application test should be made. The following procedure is a fairly safe one to follow in selecting the proper foundation shade for black skins.

Using the shade that you think most closely matches the shade of the complexion, dab a small amount onto the cheek and blend lightly. If the color begins to turn ashen, you know that the undertones, working through the foundation, have "turned" the color. Select a shade that is one tone darker. Even though it will definitely appear too dark just as you dot the face and apply it, the color will become exactly the shade desired as you blend and the undertones come through.

In cases where the color selected turns red, chances are the shade selected has too much sienna in it. Try a shade a tone lighter or one with less warmth. Yellow undertones work well with a foundation which is a cool brown, rather than a warm brown mixture.

The same basic common sense is used in the selection of foundation for black skins as for white skins. If a skin is obviously red

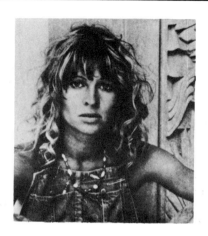

I believe in a clean, healthy look. I moisturize once a day, in the morning after washing, with a cream containing no animal fat, that I buy from a health or vegetarian shop. My favorite eyelid shade is Black Kohl—in fact, it's the only color I use! I wear it on the lid, and on the side of the eye, top and bottom. Then I put on two coats of black mascara. I never wear false eyelashes, and use only Chapstick on my lips to keep them from becoming dry. One of the first things I learned about make-up was that you must take your time putting it on!

JULIE CHRISTIE

and ruddy, you would certainly not apply a foundation with a pink overtone, etc.

There are several types of foundations: liquid, matte, whipped, cream-cake, cream-stick, cake, and medicated. The selection of the right type of foundation should depend on two factors: the skin type, and the coverage necessary or desired.

It is very important that you also realize that the coverage afforded by any one foundation is variable, depending on how heavily it is applied. In this manner, the levels of coverage are almost infinite. You might like the texture of one foundation and, with a little artistry, alter its normal coverage level or capacity.

You must always experiment. The art of make-up is not a cut-and-dried science like mathematics. In math you know that two plus two equals four, and upside down, or turned around, the same equation will bring the same result. Make-up, or rather its application, has no immutable, inflexible laws. Just as each face is different, so is the problem of enhancing each face. You must always remain flexible, inventive, and versatile.

With this in mind, the following is a **basic** description of the different types of foundation.

LIQUID: This is by far the most popular type of foundation. It is very easily applied and, depending on the manufacturer, can give anywhere from a sheer to an opaque coverage. Liquids have either a water base or an oil base, and the range of shades is very wide. They normally give the skin a glowing appearance.

MATTE: This type of foundation can come in any form, from liquid to cream to cake. The ingredient that sets the matte foundation into its own category is powder, which is mixed in as a part of its formula. Matte foundations normally give opaque coverage and give the skin a dry, dull look.

WHIPPED: A slightly heavier textured foundation than the liquid, but still, in most cases, light and frothy. It resembles whipped cream or a soufflé. Whipped foundation normally gives medium coverage. It normally has a greater amount of moisturizing qualities and leaves the skin slightly moist and glowing.

CREAM-CAKE: A condensed version of the whipped, a cream-cake is thicker and richer than any of the foundations. As directed, the application of a cream-cake foundation gives heavy screening and the most protection from dryness. The skin is given a definite creamy glow.

CREAM-STICK: Basically, the stick form is identical to a cream-cake except that it is slightly "tighter" so as to maintain its shape. The consistency is more stiff but the benefits of its coverage and its nondrying quality are the same.

CAKE: This type of foundation is rather like a dried version of the cream-cake. It is a highly compressed powder and must be applied with a wet **natural** sponge. The water and cake, when mixed together, form a paste which gives a heavy, opaque, and matte cover.

	Normal	Dry	Oily
Mild coverage	water-based liquid	oil-based liquid	water-based liquid, medicated liquid
Medium coverage	oil-based liquid	whipped	matte
Heavy coverage	whipped cream-cake	cream-cake	cake, medicated cake

MEDICATED: These are the foundations that are generally issued by a dermatologist to combat excessive oil or blemished skin. They contain antibacterial ingredients and have great astringent qualities. They come in liquid or cream, most often in tube form. Some milder medicated foundations can be purchased over the counter rather than being specifically prescribed.

Whichever foundation is selected, the proper and professional application is with a dry foam sponge rather than the fingertips, except for the cake variety, which, as described, must be applied with a wet, natural sponge.

The reasons for using a sponge are varied:

1. The sponge blends the base on much more smoothly than the fingers are able to do.
2. The sponge absorbs the excess which the fingers cannot.
3. The sponge, if kept clean and washed, will not transfer the bacteria and natural oils which the fingers transport.
4. The sponge is kinder to the delicate facial tissues than the somewhat firm fingertips.

But which type of foundation is best for which type of skin? Again, there are no immutable laws here because of the adaptability in terms of application. However, there are certain guidelines. A dry skin should not, obviously, be exposed to a drying foundation, nor an oily skin to a thick, wet cream. A highly blemished face should not wear a foundation that will cake up around each blemish, attracting even more attention, and a good complexion should not screen its healthy glow with a heavy foundation.

Basically speaking, common sense should direct you in the proper selection of a foundation type. A book can only give you so much information. You absolutely **must** get your experience from trying the make-up, feeling how it spreads, discovering the different levels of opacity it affords, and learning how it reacts.

The chart above is merely meant to give you certain very basic guidelines.

A very important factor that should be kept at the forefront of your mind is that the overall appearance of the foundation is the mainstay of the "natural look." This cosmetic fashion will probably remain forever, regardless of how many fads come and go. It is the classic cosmetic look because it is so natural, healthy-looking, and flattering!

A skin that looks artificial and unreal is considered unattractive by today's standards — and right these standards are! That is why the careful and proper application of foundation is so important. That is also why only the smallest amount of foundation, to either give one even facial tone and/or disguise imperfections of the skin, should be applied. Do not, repeat, **do not** apply more foundation than is necessary. Don't fall into that same old a-little-is-good, more-is-better routine. Normally, the less foundation you apply, the better the appearance of even troubled skin.

With the corner of your sponge, dot the face just as you did with the moisture cream, except put two or three small dots on the cheeks instead of only one. Leave the areas covered by the concealer untouched until you have carefully blended the dotted foundation all over the face. Include the eyelids and the lips. Be careful to absorb any excess from the corners of the nose and the cleft of the chin. Now, get a fresh supply of foundation by either turning the bottle over onto the sponge or dipping the corner of the sponge into the foundation. Dab the areas covered by the concealer. Remember to **dab** and not rub, push, or pull the skin. After you have dabbed the fresh supply of foundation over the concealer, turn the sponge to expose a clean corner.

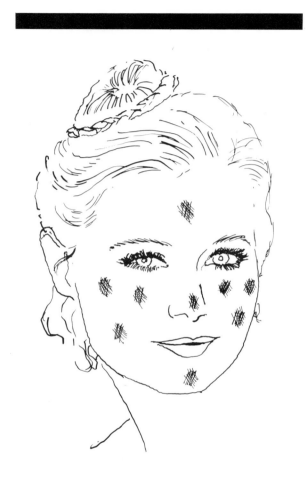

Apply foundation in dots

Continue to dab and pat this foundation exactly as you did the concealer, until you have achieved one even facial tone.

You have now created what compares to the artist's flawless canvas. Examine your efforts closely. Be objective, even downright ruthless. **Aside** from a certain polish, an all-over tone and finish, and the concealment of minor facial blemishes, does the face look made-up? Could someone guess that there is a layer of foundation on?

If so, you have either been lax in blending it evenly and carefully or you simply have applied too much!

Try again, but if you decide to wash it all off remember to follow all the necessary preliminary steps:

1. Cleanse.
2. Tone (freshener or astringent).
3. Moisturize.
4. Apply a regulator/toner if necessary.
5. Apply concealer.

This next step is to set the foundation.

APPLYING POWDER CORRECTLY

The application of a powder "sets" the foundation, which simply means keeping it fresh looking for a prolonged period. In the case of some oil-based foundations, it also means preventing it from streaking. This latter is especially important to oily skins, for the use of a well-blended powder will, to some extent, prevent the natural oils from working through the foundation.

Powdering the foundation is very important. Unfortunately, many young women do not powder because they have the mistaken notion that powdering the face is old-fashioned — something Grandma did or does. The truth is that the only old-fashioned thing about Grandma's powder was the way she put it on.

We've all seen some old ladies and, truth to tell, some young ones too who look as if they've just come from their labors in a flour mill. The powder is thick on their faces, giving their skin a dry, dusty, and artificial look. That is exactly how powder should not look!

The use of a powder puff or a cotton ball in applying loose powder makes its proper application almost impossible. All a puff or cotton ball can do is lay the powder on top of the foundation which, in most cases, completely screens the healthy glow of both the skin and the foundation.

The use of a powder brush is essential in the proper application of loose powder. Each carrying its minuscule load, the thousand bristles work the powder right **into** the foundation so that they literally become one. In place of two layers — one of foundation and one of powder — you achieve, instead, one combined film.

Some people argue that powder destroys the youthful-looking glow of the skin, and it's perfectly true that it gives the face a matte look. But that is precisely what is necessary in order to design a face of maximum attractiveness. One doesn't want total shine. Instead one wants **selective** highlights, an accent and dramatization of only **certain** areas rather than the entire face.

It is quite true that a powdered face can make age lines seem more prominent — but only if the powder is not applied correctly. That is to say, a collection of powder

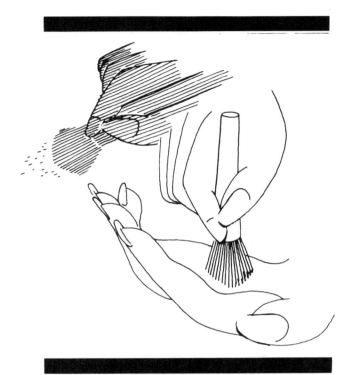

powder. Instead, brush the powder onto the skin briskly, letting the tip of each bristle work for you. The skin should feel a mild tingle from the points of the bristles rather than the soft, albeit soothing, caress of the sides of the brush.

A word here about brushes. Your end result is only as good as the tools with which you work. Good brushes will last a lifetime if you take proper care of them. So don't stint. Buy the best, and your work will reflect it.

trapped in the depression of a line is grotesquely obvious, of course. As in all steps of make-up application, **the technique is essential.**

Holding the powder brush as if it were a pencil, the tips of the bristles are dipped into the powder. In wide-mouthed containers, the brush is easily submerged. In the case of the shaker type container, a small amount of powder is shaken onto the palm of the hand, and the brush is then dipped in.

With a quick flick of the wrist, the excess powder is shaken loose from the brush. What remains on the brush is then applied to the face. The important thing is that you do not merely coat the face with a layer of the

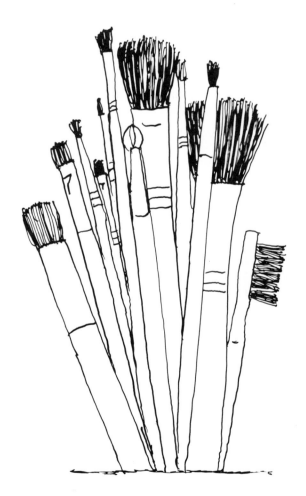

There are several types of powder. The best of these is loose **translucent** powder. Although it gives an off-white or beigy tone in the container, translucent powder has no color and, therefore, will not alter the shade of the foundation or the tone of the skin. For this reason it may be used for all shades of skin — black, white, yellow, red, etc. It is strongly recommended that this type of powder be used in doing a professional make-up.

A pressed translucent powder is available for touch-ups during the day. Pressed powder comes in compact form and is much easier to carry. The optimum method of application is with the powder brush. Many women, however, do not want to carry so much equipment around with them. In this case, a puff is acceptable for superficial touch-ups. The puff is gently dragged across the surface of the powder and then patted onto the face. To minimize the floured look, the puff should be shaken to dislodge excess powder after the initial application. Then the face is buffed with the shaken puff.

These puffs must be kept scrupulously clean. Not only will an excess of powder accumulate, making proper application impossible, but the natural oils from the face and fingers, which are absorbed by the puff, will turn rancid. These rancid oils (and any collected dirt), when pushed onto the face, can cause blemishes and give off a sour aroma.

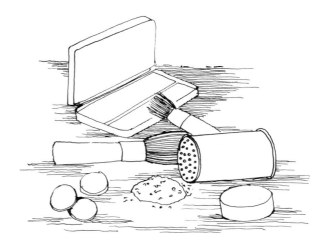

Another type of powder is called **iridescent** or **pearlized** powder. It is a powder of the types described above with the addition of an iridescent ingredient. This type of powder gives the face an all-over luminous look.

There are also tinted face powders. These come in a variety of shades and are intended to be worn either without any foundation or to augment or intensify the applied foundation.

If there is anything old-fashioned about powder, it is this tinted type. Many women, and some professional make-up artists, however, like using them. You should experiment and see if you like the effect they create. For the proper selection, choose a slightly lighter tint than that of the foundation. The same color will intensify the shade and a darker one will, obviously, make the skin look deeper in tone. You can also experiment with pink, green, white and mauve tinted powders to achieve different pigmentation corrections such as the toners achieve.

Whichever type of powder is used, it should be applied artfully so that it is not apparent to the observing eye. It is also important that it is well blended, and particular attention must be paid to the eyelids, the sides of the nose, and the areas covered by the concealer. If it looks like the face is covered with powder, there is either too much on or it has not been blended in well enough.

Your flawless canvas has now been totally prepared, and you are ready, like that old lyric, to "accentuate the positive and eliminate the negative."

PERFECTING YOUR BROW

It is a good practice to get into the habit of working downward on the face. It saves a lot of time otherwise spent in touching-up what has already been made-up. In other words, if you begin your artistry on the brows and finish your make-up application at the lips, your hands or tools will not be constantly going over already made-up areas. In this way you save the time necessary for any possible touch-ups.

The brows are an important feature of the face. Many women neglect to consider them in this light. They convey moods and expressions, but, most important, they frame the eyes. Since the eyes are the most outstanding feature of the face, they can reflect an unbalanced expression if they are not framed properly. Just as a cartoonist can effect a startled look of surprise by

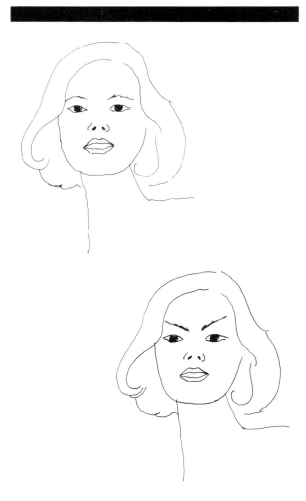

Expressions altered by brow shapes

drawing two high semicircles over the eyes or a look of seething anger by the use of two diagonal lines, so can the shape of the brow affect what expression is transmitted. Moreover, just as you would not frame a painting with inappropriate molding, so should you evaluate and design the brows to balance and enhance the eyes.

Classically speaking, the brows should begin directly above the inside corner of the eye, rise into a natural arch over the outer edge of the iris, gently decline, and end at the point diagonally above the outer corner of the eye.

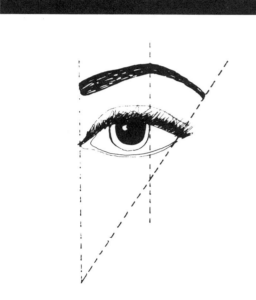

Classic brow alignment

To measure accurately, hold a pencil at the side of the nose, lining it up with the inside corner of the eye. That is the spot where the brow should begin. Now move the pencil so that it touches the side of the nostril and the outer corner of the eye. This is where the brow should end. Looking straight into the mirror, the high point of the arch should be directly above the outer edge of the iris.

Naturally, all these evaluations should be made before applying any make-up.

Practically everybody needs corrective tweezing and this should, obviously, be done before any cosmetics are applied to the face.

The classic shape, as described above, can be adapted to a variety of fashion looks — pencil thin, slightly thicker, wider at the inner corner, etc. The essential judgment should **not** be based on the type of brow preferred but on the type of brow that would be best for the features of the face. Again, there are no hard and fast rules about one shape brow versus another shape. This is something which is developed with experience. However, a pencil thin brow on a big-boned, large-nosed face would accentuate rather then subtract from its heavy, overbearing appearance. Tiny semicircular brows on wide-eyed, round faces would create an even more round and full look. Common sense must always be used regardless of any fashion trend.

There are a variety of tweezers available: blunt edge, wedge shaped, rounded point. Most popular are the wedge shaped. However, the rounded point tweezers are good to have as a standby pair for certain uses. After measuring and evaluating the shape of brow most suitable, you may want to wipe the brow area with a liquid pain deadener. Anbesol is recommended for use on the gums, but it is also handy in softening the annoying pain of tweezing. There are several other painkillers available without prescription for external use. Otherwise, a moisture cream softens the skin and therefore makes the tweezing less painful.

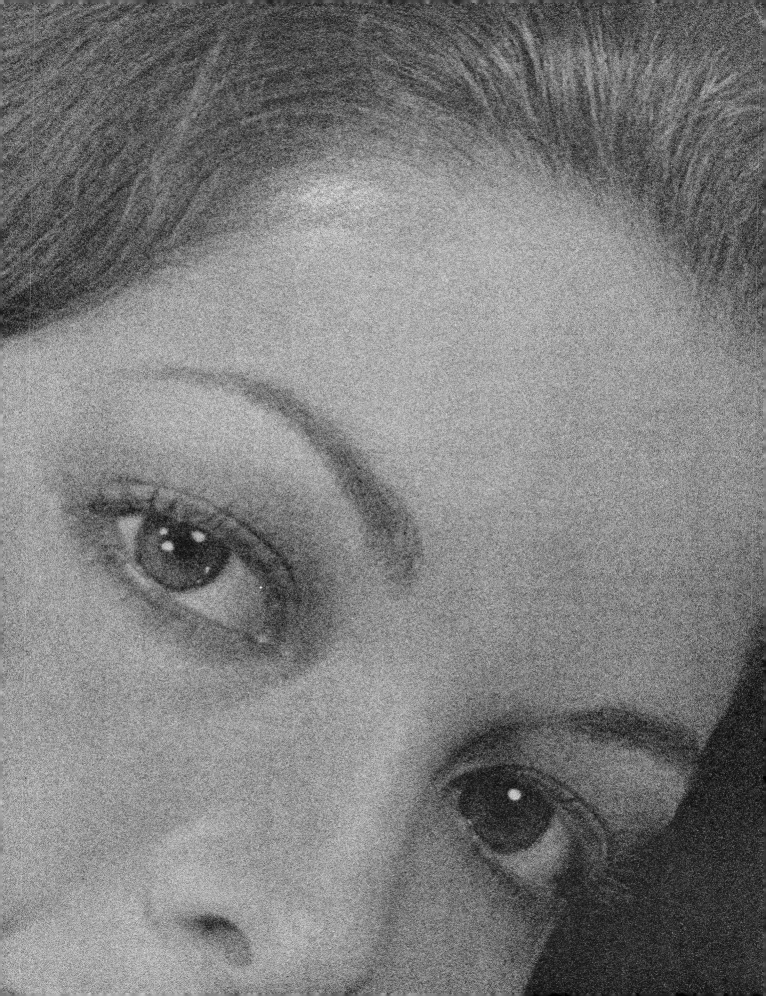

Hold the skin firmly, stretching it between the thumb and the index finger. One by one, pluck each unwanted hair in the direction in which it grows. Always pluck from the underside of the brow. In all cases you want to make as much room between the brow and the lash as possible. In very few cases will you have to remove any hair from above, other than a straggler or two.

Do one brow at a time and proceed carefully and slowly. If you are unsure as to whether or not a particular hair should be removed, pull it away from the brow without plucking it. Judge whether or not it leaves a sparse space or whether it helps to define the brow shape. One by one, continue tweezing until the shape has been established. Then wipe the brow with a little witch hazel or alcohol (or your skin toner) and proceed to the second brow.

A word here about the symmetry of the brows. You will, of course, try to make each brow the same as the other. In most cases, however, the brows, themselves, are different; the hair grows in different directions or the shape is slightly different. Do not become alarmed if, hair for hair, each brow is not an exact duplicate of the other. The very slight difference is one of the things that gives us individuality.

The shape or size of the brow can be altered by using certain fool-the-eye techniques employed to correct eyes that are too closely set or too widely set. To offset the closely set eye, expand the brow by

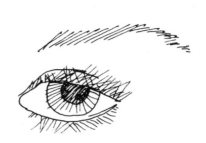

Brow shape for closely set eye

starting it at a point slightly beyond the inside corner of the eye and extending it slightly beyond the outer corner. This gives the illusion that the eyes are more widely spaced. Widely spaced eyes are more rare, but they can be enhanced by beginning the brows closer to each other and ending them farther in from the temples.

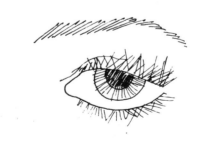

Brow shape for widely set eye

43

How does one judge whether the eye is too widely set, too closely set, or just right? Classically speaking, the eyes should be separated by the width of one eye.

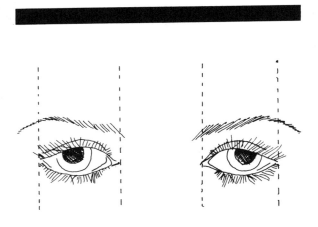

Perfectly spaced eyes

Sometimes tweezing is not enough. Sometimes the hair is too sparse and the desired shape is not naturally there, just waiting to be defined. In these cases one must **fill in** the brows to create the desired shape. Filling in is accomplished via two mediums: the eyebrow pencil or a powder shadow (sometimes called "brush-on brow").

The pressed shadow is easier to use and gives a soft, natural look. The pencil requires more craft but can give the appearance of real eyebrows when used properly. A combination of both mediums may be used to really fool the observing eye.

The powder shadow is applied with a small, wedge-shaped brush. Holding the brush as one would a pencil, a small amount of the powder is transported to the brow and gently brushed onto the skin in tiny hairlike strokes to the shape desired. Another brush, called a **brow brush,** is employed to soften the effect. This is done by brushing over the applied powder, which removes some of it and creates a mottled appearance.

The pencil is slightly more difficult. A fine point must always be maintained and, with this point, tiny hairlike lines are meticulously drawn onto the skin in the desired shape. Each little line is drawn in the same direction that the hair it is replacing, or rather imitating, would grow. These little hairlike lines should exactly resemble the surrounding hairs in color and in texture. A brow brush is then gently passed over these drawn hairs to soften the effect.

In certain cases you may want to use both techniques. You may want to put a soft background of powder down and then pencil in some hairlike lines. This gives the brows a super natural, genuine look. In the case of matching or duplicating frosted or bleached hair, select a powder shadow that is of the lighter hue and a pencil to

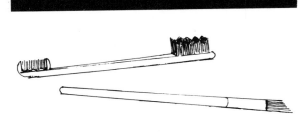

Brow brush/comb and #4 wedge

represent the darker tone. Gray or salt-and-pepper brows are especially attractive with this technique.

Many times the natural brows are too dark. They are overbearing and give the face a hard look. In these cases, the brows should be bleached. There are products on the market that have been designed specifically for the layman's use and are safer for do-it-yourselfers than the more powerful bleaches used in beauty salons by professional hairdressers. That does not mean that the directions of these milder versions should not be followed precisely. To see the effect, or for day-to-day lightening, it is possible to temporarily lighten the brows with the use of creams and pastes. This method is not as effective as the bleach but is still very useful.

An off-white cream is lightly brushed onto the brow with a stiff brush such as a #4 wedge. The brows are then **combed** with a fine-toothed comb to free them from excessive cream. The comb is run through the brows several times until the brow assumes a natural salt-and-pepper look.

The brows remain lightened until you remove the cream with your cleanser. This system is particularly good for judging whether or not the brows are more effective when lightened.

There are also brow-setting lotions available. These lotions act much like a hair spray, except that they are brushed on instead of being sprayed on. The liquid is applied with a soft brush, saturating the brow. The stiffer brow brush is then em-

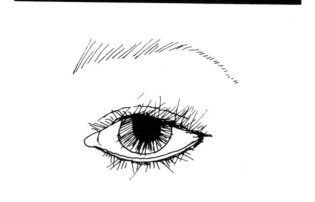

Sophia Loren-type brow

ployed to arrange the hairs in the desired shape, and the lotion "sets" the brow in place.

This setting lotion is particularly handy for long, straggly brows but is altogether essential for the Sofia Loren type brow — that is, each hair being brushed upward instead of lying horizontally.

A glycerine soap, petroleum jelly (Vaseline), or the careful and scant application of transparent lash glue also works well to set the brow into any desired shape.

THE EYE

Your attention can now be drawn to the eye itself. It has already been said, but it bears repeating: The eyes are, or should be, the most outstanding feature of the face. It is through the eyes that people express anger, kindness, sympathy, mirth, boredom, and so forth ad infinitum. You have heard it time and time again: "She's not very pretty but she has lovely eyes," or "She wouldn't be half as pretty without those big eyes."

The eyes are the focal point of the face — they are the objects people look into while speaking or trying to evaluate an impression or mood. They are the "windows of the soul."

In professional make-up, great care is taken to make sure that the eyes **are** the focal point of the face; the feature that one notices first. The eyes are also the first area where the art of cosmetic sculpturing is employed.

Cosmetic sculpturing is the use of highlighting and contouring. With reference to what has already been written about the principle of light and dark, highlighting colors are those that are light and bright, while contouring colors are those that are dark or dull. This is not as simple as it may seem. Remember that this principle is a relative one. Although an off-white color may seem at first to be a highlighting color, it is not at all **if** it is placed next to a pure white. It then becomes the contouring color — follow? For this reason, there are no unbreakable rules nor any charts that have any significance when it comes to dividing highlighters and contours. Perhaps the simplest method of evaluating these shades is to engrave the following into your mind: A highlighting color is one which is **lighter** than the surrounding colors. A contour is just the opposite — any color which is **darker** than the surrounding colors. Another graven image should be that, working together, a contour and highlighter create a perfect marriage. Although they are both effective when used alone, it is only when they are used concur-

rently that the full power of their combined magic is truly demonstrated.

Make a simple test for yourself. Look at something black. Now look at something white. Now put the two colors together. Isn't it true that the black looks much blacker when placed next to the white, and vice versa?

It is for this reason that whenever a highlighter is employed, a contour should be applied right next to it for greater definition and emphasis — this, of course, with an artful, experienced hand.

The purpose of cosmetic sculpturing in the area of the eye is: to dramatize that which nature has already constructed; to correct it optically, whenever possible; and to offer the observing eye a more structured and defined focal point.

Because the observer finds shaped planes much more interesting than flat ones, the professional make-up artist accentuates these configurations. The brow bone is generally highlighted; the crease or hollow of the eyelid is, normally, contoured; the lid is accentuated.

The "perfect" eye is solely and strictly in the eye of the beholder. There is no supreme judge to declare and acclaim Jane Fonda's eye, for instance, more perfect than Barbra Streisand's — or Donald Duck's, for that matter. This is something that is personal and is developed by studying faces, the shape of the features, the line, balance, and composition. Only then can you arrive at your own educated conclusions of what your ideal, **your** perfect eye is. Until that time, the only ground rule that can possibly be given is that the natural fold of the eyelid should lie just about one-third of the way between the brows and the lashes.

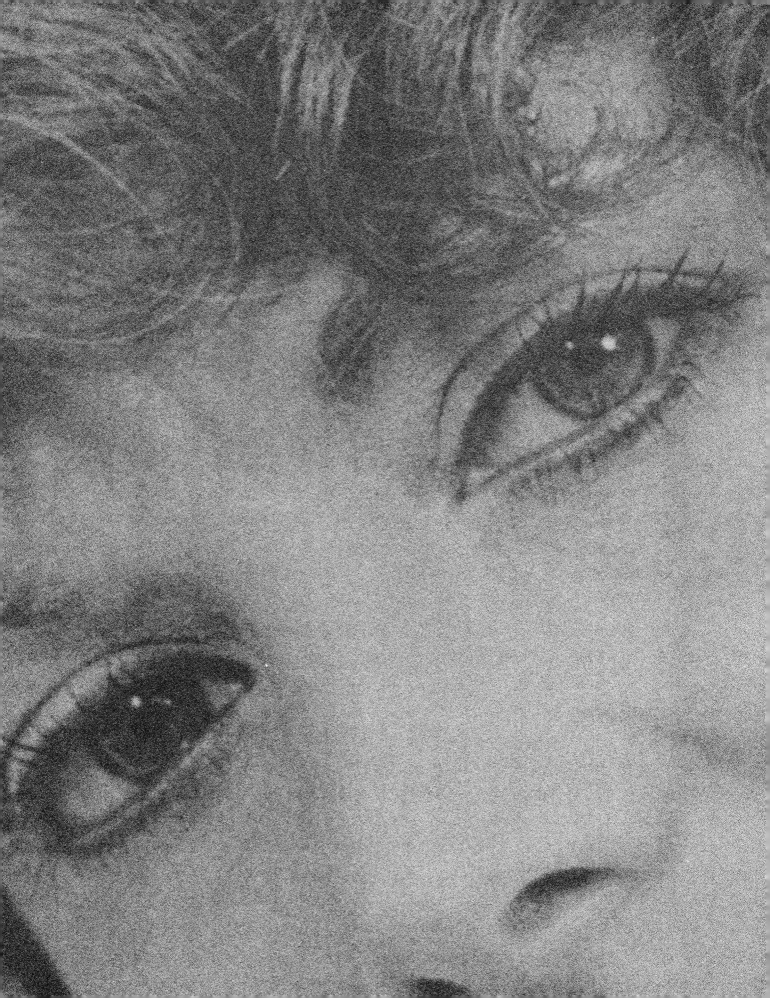

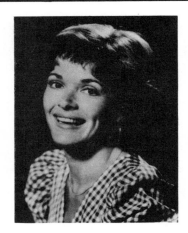

I've learned to make my make-up look soft and natural. I use a cream eyeshadow in a wine shade, and brown eye contour color with white for highlight. Then I put on eyeliner and two coats of mascara in brown, not black. Thank God for my eyes or my face would be a disaster. (The one feature of my face I've always hated was my nose.) I use a cream foundation in a shade that matches my complexion. I highlight my cheekbones and contour my face (forehead, cheek hollows, and chin) with a cream bronze-tone rouge. My favorite color lipstick is Different Sherry, by Clinique. And lipgloss is a must!

JESSICA WALTER

Professional eye make-up is generally made up of three, sometimes four, color zones and the same amount of color tones: the lid color, the contour color, the highlight color, and sometimes, the super-highlight color.

The lid color is applied from corner to corner, from the root of the lash up to the contour color. Sometimes this color is also extended down to the lower lash.

The contour color is applied in a natural-looking, shadow-imitating, soft line along the natural crease or fold of the lid.

The highlighting color is applied to the area directly beneath the brows down to the contour color.

The super-highlight is applied only when added emphasis is needed for greater distance between brow and lash. It is applied directly under the inside brow, down to the contour color.

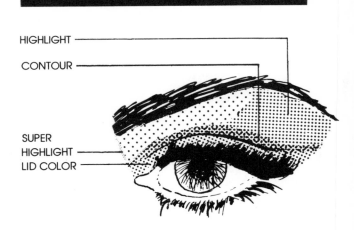

Eyeshadow color zones

The above directions are given for use on a "normal" eye that needs no corrective measures. They are very rare.

More often, the contour line must be applied to the area slightly above the natural fold of the eye. This is done for two reasons: Either the lid needs expanding, or the brow bone is too low and close to the lid. Another, and more important, reason is in the treatment of the deeply set eye.

Follow the principle. If an existing, natural shadow is brushed with a contour color, what would happen? Yes, the shadow would appear to increase in depth and therefore optically recede. Obviously, a **deeply set eye** should not be contoured directly on the natural fold of the lid, as that would create the illusion that the eye was even more deeply set. Therefore, what is needed is the creation of another "natural" fold, an optical illusion that will fool the observing eye into thinking that the real indentation is higher.

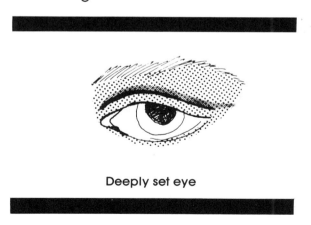

Deeply set eye

This is accomplished by applying a light-colored eyeshadow to the lid from corner to corner and from the root of the lashes into the natural fold and beyond, up

into the new contour line. This new contour line should follow the natural one, but should be placed slightly above it, in most cases, directly on the brow bone that is creating the deep socket.

The highlighter is then applied just below the brow and down to the new contour.

Supporting and emphasizing each other, the highlight color makes the contour color more effective, and vice versa. The brow bone that is highlighted is optically projected. The new contoured zone seems to recede even more because it is next to the projecting area. The lid area, including the disguised natural fold, is projected forward because of the light-colored eyeshadow and because of its position directly next to an area that is optically recessed.

It is extremely important that you understand this principle. Without it, you can never hope to master the art of professional make-up. It is, therefore, recommended that you review and study, experiment and test, over and over again, until the concept is reflexive.

Give yourself a little test now. The deeply set eye was discussed above. How would you treat the opposite type of eye, the protruding or **bulging eye**? Do not read on until you have mentally outlined your approach.

If you said, "Highlight the brow bone slightly, only to accentuate its configuration; contour with a deep tone either along the natural fold or, if need be, slightly above it; and then place a medium-dark shade on the lid," you would be perfectly correct. If you did not think along those line, please stop now and reevaluate. Do not go on until you have mastered the concept of how light colors reflect and dark colors absorb. How light colors give the illusion of filling out a depression and how dark colors make these same depressions seem more profound. How, given a perfectly flat surface, a light color applied in a straight line down the middle will make the flat area seem bowed in the middle, versus a dark line placed in the middle, which will give the illusion of a concave surface.

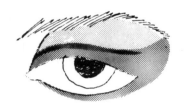

Bulging eye

Those of you who immediately understood the concept are probably saying, "Alright, already!" But a review **is** necessary because the principle is so important.

The **small eye** is treated by applying a light-colored eyeshadow on the lid, from the root of the lash up to the contour color and from the inside corner of the eye out beyond the outside corner. The highlight

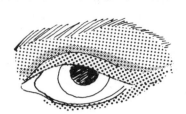

Small eye

color is applied to the area directly below the brow and down to the contour color.

Closely set eyes can be optically separated by applying all the eye make-up as you would with a normal eye except you start at a point away from the corner of the eye.

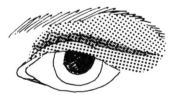

Closely set eye

Widely set eyes should really be treated exactly as normal eyes. They are regarded, by Greek standards, as the most beautiful of all. However, as with most singular characteristics, women who are blessed with them unfortunately tend to yearn for the more average. If widely set eyes are to look more closely set, the application of all

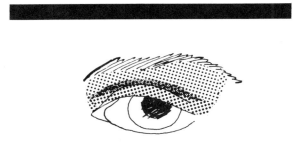

Widely set eye

three of the tones should be placed closer to the nose.

This seems to be an appropriate time to discuss individuality. An individuality is something that sets a person apart from the norm. A birthmark, a mole, a hooked nose. All of these may seem unattractive characteristics, something to camouflage — **if** you want to look like everybody else. Arlene Dahl, who was voted one of the ten most beautiful women in the world, uses a mole near her upper lip as her trademark. Barbra Streisand's hooked nose is hardly the normal, everyday movie star's wish fulfillment.

This is an age of individualism. This is an age when the standards for a pretty face are not simply based on "cheerleader prettiness." An unusual face is hailed as being beautiful, an ugly face as interesting. There is absolutely no reason, today, for any woman to be unattractive!

Getting back to the eye. Study it in relation to the face and the important role it plays. If it's small, should it be made to look bigger, or is it, somehow, strangely attractive as it is? Do your deeply set eyes look like two holes, or can you make them look like the proverbial deep pools? In other words, don't strive for a uniform look. Try to make that face outstanding in the crowd.

There are several types of eyeshadows with which to create any effect you wish. There are powders, creams, cream sticks, gels, pencils, and liquids. It is impossible to say one is better than the other. They each have characteristics that have varied appeal.

The powder shadow generally lasts the longest. It is applied with a brush or a felt-tipped applicator and comes in the widest range of colors. Contrary to what many women think, powder shadow does not affect or cause dry skin. Some powder shadows may be applied either wet or dry. The wet application intensifies the color.

Cream shadow comes in a variety of textures. The color in the package is very seldom exactly the shade after application, because cream shadows tend to dissipate, somewhat, in blending. Most creams ultimately form a grease line on the lid just about on the natural crease. This can be allieviated, to some extent, by careful powdering. There **are** creams, however, that do not dissipate and do not form this crease. These are clearly marked so as to announce this great advantage. Creams may be applied with a felt-tipped applicator, a brush, or the fingertip. The latter is the least acceptable as the finger can hardly reach into all the small angles.

A cream stick is a slightly sturdier cream shadow that is molded into a stick form,

51

resembling a thin lipstick. They come in miniature lipsticklike tubes, in paper-covered crayons, or in wood-cased pencils. The sticks are soft, the crayons softer, the wood-encased pencils softest. That is to say, ideally, how they **should** be. However, standards vary from manufacturer to manufacturer. Again, you must experiment with products from as many sources as possible until you find the tone and texture you prefer.

Gel eyeshadows are sometimes packaged in little tubs but are generally put on the market in tube form. They either dry on the lid and form the same crease line later on as do the creams, or they dry on the lid with a wet look. This wet look resembles the cream eyeshadow freshly applied, but, unlike the cream, is dry to the touch.

The liquid eyeshadow is painted on with a brush and dries matte, much like eyeliner.

There is no reason for maintaining the same type of eyeshadow throughout the eye make-up application. If you like, you may use any type for any zone: powder on the lid, cream for the crease, a gel for the highlight. No one will take you to court for mixing. You must, however, know your medium. Before you blithely apply a mixture to the lid area, make sure you've experimented enough to know what kind of reaction to expect.

In terms of precedence, again, there

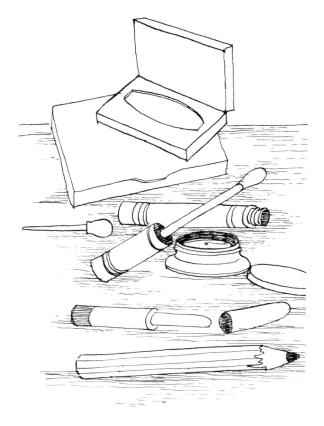

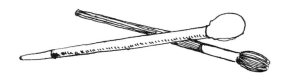

are no hard and fast rules. For the beginner, it is much easier to apply the contour shadow first. This clearly outlines exactly where the two other zones will lie. It is also less confusing to the inexperienced eye to either measure halfway or to discern the exact placement for corrective techniques. In any case, one shadow should blend softly into the other, leaving no line of demarcation between the two, and leaving no bare skin, either.

The use of a super-highlighter is solely for exaggerated expansion. If the brow is too close to the eye, if the lid is too completely hidden — in short, wherever bolder measures are necessary. This super-highlighter is not used extensively. It is solely used to high-light the highlight.

The selection of the **ideal** colors for the eye is very important, too. Unfortunately, there is not (and cannot ever be) one simple chart to outline exactly what color should be applied to what color eye. There are just too many variables. There are, however, certain factors that can be considered as constant. The first rule, if there be one, is that eye make-up is applied for the **sole** reason of enhancing the eyes. It's prime purpose is to make the eyes look more beautiful. It is not applied so that the costume, the dress, the shirt, the sweater will look prettier. No, simply and purely, without question, it is applied for the sole benefit of the eyes. (It follows naturally that when the eyes look good, the face looks better.)

For that reason, the color of the eyeshadows selected must be chosen sole-ly for the effect they will have upon the eyes. Therefore, blue eyes will, of course, be enhanced by the use of blue shadow. Green eyes by green. Brown eyes by green, turquoise, etc. That does not mean that blue eyes should **always** wear blue eyeshadow. Nor does it stop there.

You must consider the depth of color as well as the shade because it, too, affects what color the iris will reflect. A pale blue eye will seem shades lighter and cooler if a Wedgwood blue or navy blue eyeshadow is applied to the lid. The same blue eye will seem much darker if a shade of eyeshadow much lighter than the iris is applied. By the same token, a hazel eye will appear much greener with the application of a medium-toned, yellowish green eyeshadow, while a blue shadow will make the same eye look warm brown.

It's the same principle of light and dark: The dark eyeshadow makes the light eye seem lighter **by comparison**, and vice versa. So, you must consider not only what color will enhance the eye but also what shade of that color.

That is not to say that there is one, and only one, shade per set of eyes. If that were true there would not be the ever increasing range of colors that is available. There is, though, a prime color for a particular pur-pose. It is rather difficult to learn exactly which are these optimum colors except through experimentation and through study of the color wheel. Through use of this wheel you can learn what colors go into making other colors. In this way you can learn which colors accentuate each other and which minimize.

As far as the choice of the proper color combinations to create the different zones of eye make-up is concerned, the only rule is that these colors should harmonize. You may prefer the **one color family**, i.e., three different blues, or three greens, or three vi-olets. Or you may find that combinations of colors are more effective. In either event, the one hard rule is that they be broken up into three (and sometimes four) different and distinct intensities:

1. The dark tone   the contour
2. The medium tone   the lid color
3. the light tone   the highlighter
4. The lightest tone   the super-highlighter

There are certain irregularities that exist with reference to certain eyeshadows. They are outlined here because they are fairly constant, but you should definitely experiment yourself so that you can practice a discerning eye when it comes to judging these quirks.

Normally, a blue-eyed, fair-skinned woman can wear a blue eyeshadow very well and have it enhance her looks. Some women, however, have very fine, thin skin through which blood vessels and veins are apparent. This type of skin does not take blue shadows well as they pick up the blueness of the veins, making the skin look faintly blue all over.

Some hazel-eyed girls have olive complexions. Normally, their eyes would be enhanced by the use of a green eyeshadow. The green, however, magnifies the green or yellow tinge to their skin. This can, of course, be corrected somewhat by rouge, lipstick, and the proper foundation, but it is a factor to be reckoned with.

Then again, some eyes are somewhat shot with tiny capillaries. These give the whites of the eyes a reddish (bloodshot) appearance. The red that is combined with blue to make a violet or purple eyeshadow will accentuate this redness. It is not, therefore, the wisest choice, to select a violet, mauve, or pink eyeshadow for this type of eye.

As you experiment, you will find irregularities of your own. The more you do, the more you'll come to acknowledge that there are no firm, unbendable canons when it comes to the art of make-up.

The same holds true to the applicators used in applying make-up. Each artist has a favorite brush for a particular area. The numbers and types of brushes used in the eye area are varied. The following is a brief outline to help you begin your own explorations.

	POWDER	CREAM	GEL
Contour shadow	"fluff" or round #8 soft	#4 wedge	#4 round
Lid color	#6 or #8 flat	#6 or #8 flat	"fluff" or #8 round
Highlight	#4 flat	#6 or #4 flat	#4 round

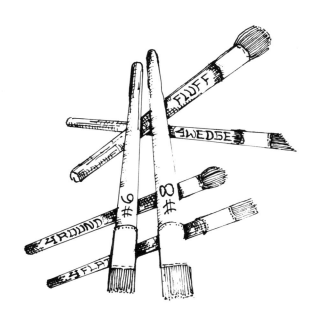

The pencils, sticks, and crayons are applied directly and blended with a fingertip. There are cases, however, when the fingertip is too wide to do an adequate job. The use of a brush or felt-tipped applicator is then recommended.

Fashion trends in eye make-up come and go. Obviously, you will want to keep abreast of these fashions and experiment with them. It is important that you do so. However, the eye make-up that is outlined above is classic and its principles can always be maintained.

There are, however, other fashionably chic eye make-ups that may do even more for your appearance. These make-ups are basically designed more for their glamour value than for the pure enhancement of the eye but, in some cases, they draw attention and convert what can be an average or plain face into one of more interest — if they are done discreetly and with discernment. Too much make-up or the grotesque application of it serves only one purpose: to make the observer critically aware that its the kind of beauty that so easily rubs off with a damp cloth.

Look at the fashion magazines and analyze the models' make-up. Try to duplicate some of the layouts, the plans, for their make-up application but don't apply as much depth of color as do they. In other words, subdue that which you see. Remember that models in photographs can carry off a more bizarre look just by the very nature of their work and the demands of it. In almost every case, models on the street do not wear all the make-up they have on in the editorial pages. But do copy the angles and the areas of application, then look at yourself as critically as possible for an honest evaluation. Better yet, have a Polaroid taken or go to your nearest twenty-five-cent photo machine. Sometimes you just can't see yourself "in the flesh," and the two-dimensional reflection shows you what the observer sees. (Don't go out and shoot yourself afterward. The lighting, etc., plays an important role and you can rest assured that you don't always look that bad! If, however, you look good in a low quality photo such as that, go right out and list yourself with the police — you're dangerous!)

After you've mastered handling the brushes and the classic eye make-up already described, you might like to try another very good basic (if not yet classic) treatment. This is only recommended for those who have a visible eyelid area when the eye is completely open. Select what would normally be the contour color — a brown, a Wedgwood, a gray, something somewhat medium in tone — and apply it from corner to corner, incorporating the contour area as well. Leave a narrow path directly over the iris, from the root of the lash up to the contour color. Blend the combined lid/contour color up over the last fourth of the brow bone, the area at the outside corner which would normally be covered with the highlight color. Now highlight the unshadowed narrow path of the eyelid and the remaining area directly beneath the beginning of the brow down to the contour. Use a fairly light color. With a fingertip or with a clean brush, carefully blend the

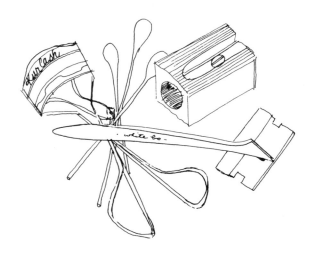

darker shades in the corners emphasize the depth, the highlight color in the very center of the lid brings the impact of the planes into focus.

You are now at the point where greater intensification of the eye area is achieved by **rimming**. (This is not lining, which will be discussed later.) Don't mistake this rimming as a step to be followed after the last-described eye make-up only. This is a basic step that would be followed at all times.

Most every eye can use some further intensification via the use of pencils on the rims of the eye. The area I refer to is the flat, moist surface closest to the eyeball. This area serves as an ideal arena for persuading the observer to see that which we prefer to be seen.

You can make your eyes look bigger by applying a white to the lower rim. The observer interprets this white as part of the whites of the eyes, which optically creates a larger eye. The use of a pale blue line on the lower rim makes the eye whites look whiter.

The application is quite simple, if somewhat ticklish. Using a grease pencil that has been warmed by rolling the tip between your thumb and index finger or one of the newer soft eyeshadow pencils, follow the line of your inside rims. This can be more easily accomplished by pulling the lid down and away from your eyeball with one hand while you skim the surface of the rim with the pencil held in the other. For application on the upper rim, use your index finger to pull the eyelid up and away from the eyeball. Carefully skim the exposed surface, making sure that the pencil's tip is not too sharp.

eyeshadows so that all the edges of the color zones are flowing into each other and you cannot see a definite demarcation. It's important, however, that in blending you do not carry the darker tone onto the lighter tone.

Don't be intimidated if it looks a little bizarre at first. Anything new looks a little exotic until you are familiar with it. The only thing to be concerned with is the proper blending of the colors. The purpose of this type of eye make-up is to accentuate the round structure of the eyeball while maintaining the contoured structure as well. The

Below is a list of tricks these pencils can achieve.

1. Make eyes look bigger by applying white or off-white to the lower rim. If your upper rim is visible, applying the white or off-white to the upper rim will further increase the optical illusion.
2. Make blue eyes seem darker and bluer by applying light blue, make the same eyes look paler by applying a darker blue.
3. Make blue eyes seem violet by using a violet pencil.
4. Make green eyes greener by applying a dark, forest green or a yellow.
5. Make blue eyes look clear, icy blue by applying forest or kelly green.
6. Make the whites of the eyes seem whiter and clearer with light blue.
7. Make dark eyes seem darker with violet.
8. Make the eyes seem to sparkle with silver.
9. Safely duplicate the sultry mystery of kohl with black.
10. Augment the fullness of the lashline by applying black to the upper rim.
11. Try charcoal gray on the lower rim, with black on the upper rim, for a glamorous eye.

We now arrive at the controversial eyeliner. By some standards, eyeliner is superfluous and dated. Unfortunately, no matter how passé eyeliner may be in relation to current fashion trends, some women **need** it! Just as in any other trend, you must evaluate and judge for yourself that which is best for you.

The purpose of eyeliner is to define the eye and give it greater clarity and structure. As luck would have it, some eyes do not need this clarification. For them there is no controversy. For those eyes that **do** need it, however, the advice is to use it — but use it well.

Eyeliner should always match the shade of the lashes. In this way it can give the illusion of thicker lashes and can also work to discreetly alter the shape of the eye, when that deception is necessary.

If preferred, it can also become part of the lid-contour-highlight trio. In these cases, it should harmonize with those colors. For basic application, a fine line drawn from the inner corner of the eye to the outer corner adds greater definition to any eye.

The important factor in applying a basic lining is the correct applicator. The brush must be but a few hairs wide. A #00 is ideal for this purpose. Practice using this brush until you feel you can control it easily. See how the harder the pressure on the brush, the wider the line it draws.

Since you want to achieve the finest line possible, you'll want to learn to control the brush with a featherweight touch. Start your line just about where the lashes grow. Holding the brush as if it were a pencil, and pulling the lid taut at the outer corner, lightly apply a fine line close to the lash root. Do not leave any bare skin between the lashes and the line but, rather, get the tiny tip of the brush down to the point right above the lashes. Draw this line out to the end of the lashes.

5   Dot the face with foundation.
Blend, using a dry foam sponge.

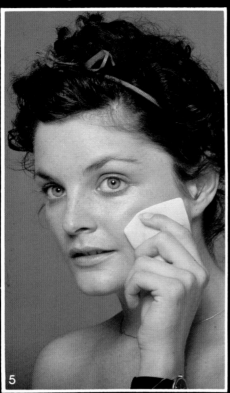

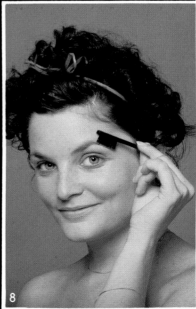

6   Notice how the application of
the foundation provides one even
facial tone. Be careful to blend so
that no lines of demarcation are
visible.

7   Apply translucent powder with a
Powder brush.

8   Using a brow brush, shape the
brows while freeing them from any
clinging powder.

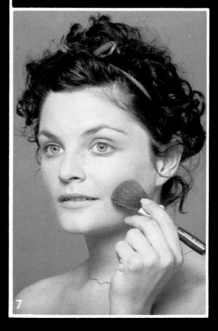

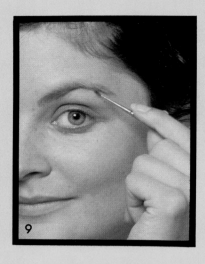

9 Fill in the brows using a #4 Wedge brush and powder shadow.

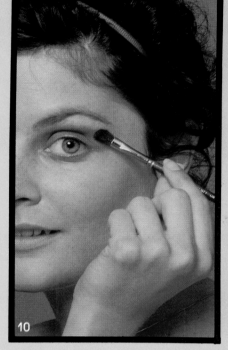

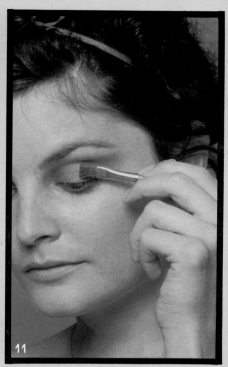

10 Accentuate the contour of the eye using a Fluff brush and the selected shadow.

11 Apply the lid color with a #8 brush.

12 Notice how the shadow is blended to avoid any hard lines of demarcation.

13 Using a #6 brush, bring the color down along the roots of the lower lash.

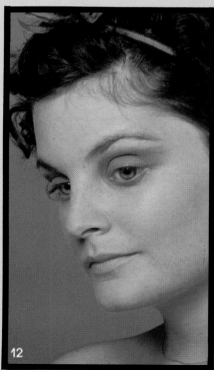

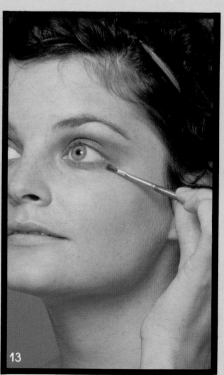

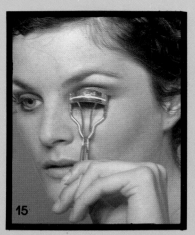

15

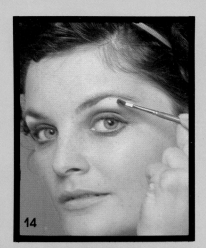

14

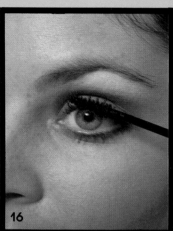

16

14   With a clean # 6 brush, apply the highlight color under the brows.

15   Carefully curl the lashes.

16   Apply mascara to both the upper and the lower lashes.

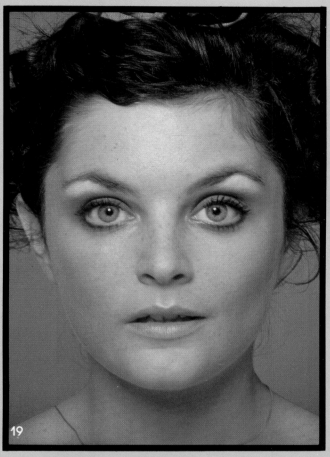

19

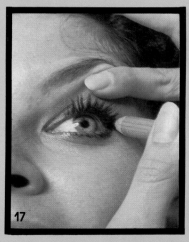

17

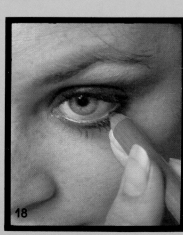

18

17   Line the upper inside rim,

18   as well as the lower inside rim, using a soft pencil shadow.

19   The completed eye make-up should dramatize the eye attractively.

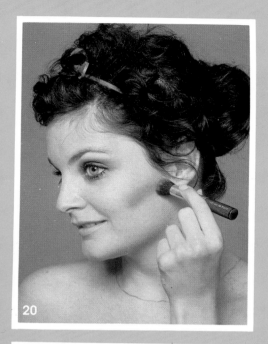

20

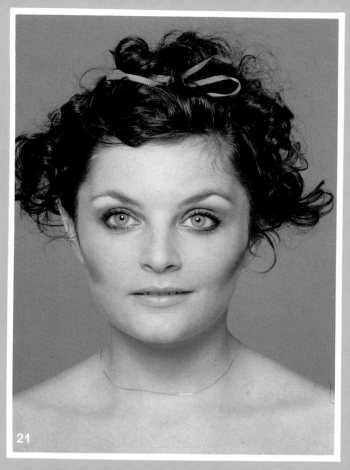

21

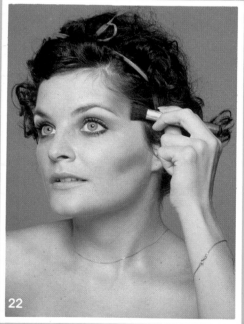

22

20 Define the cheekbones by applying contour color with a Contour brush.

21 See how this color optically increases the lift of the bone. (Compare with # 19)

22 If necessary, further increase the bone structure by contouring the temples.

23 Notice how these areas are shaded before being blended to look like natural shadows.

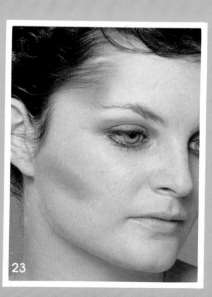

23

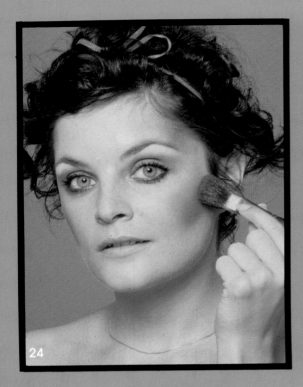

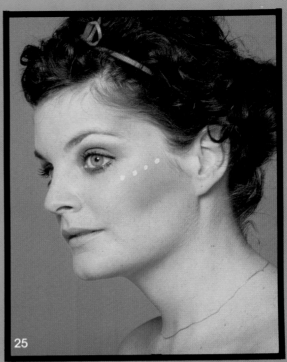

24 Cheek color is applied with a Rouge brush, blending carefully so that this color merges with the contour color, leaving no line of demarcation between the two.

25 Dot the crest of the cheekbone with a highlighter.

26 Blend carefully to avoid any hard lines.

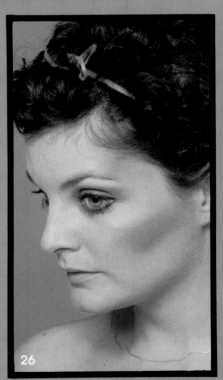

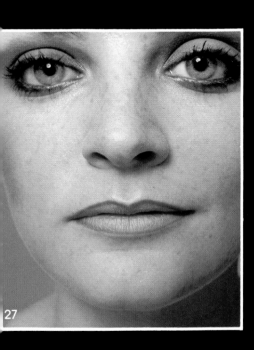

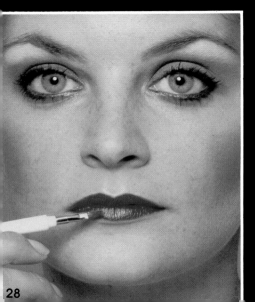

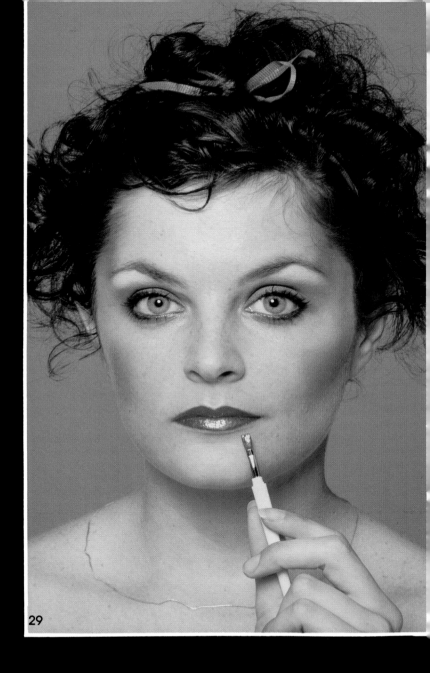

27 Outline the lips using a pointed lip pencil.

28 Fill in with a lip brush and lipstick.

29 Add a touch of lipgloss with the lip brush to intensify the lustre.

30 A d admire the finished product!

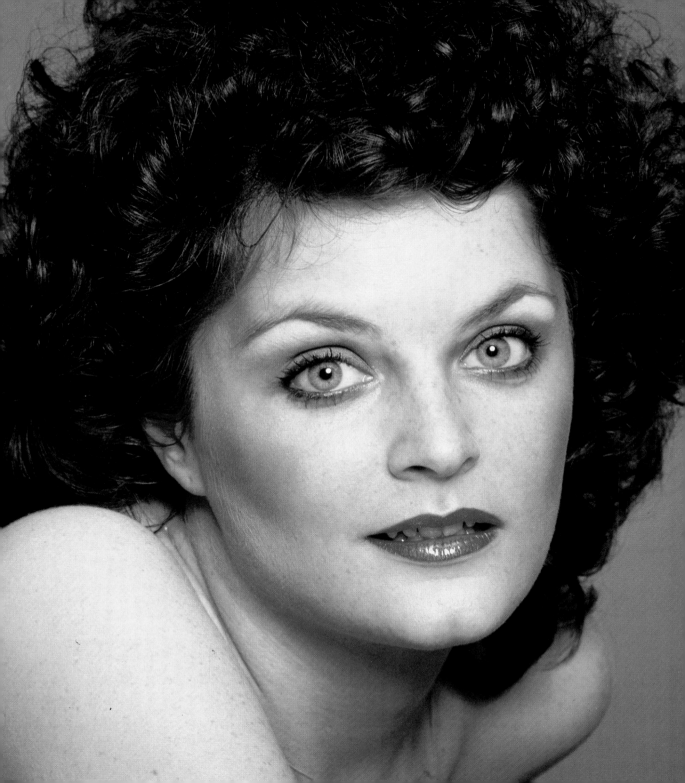

Another method for the intensification of the eye is the smudged eyeline. This is eyelining that is not so readily observable. It is applied with either a soft eyeshadow pencil or a normal eyeshadow (powder or cream). I do not recommend the usual eyeliner pencil unless it is very soft and greasy, enabling the line it draws to be smudged without leaving any hard lines. The area of coverage is identical to the classic eyelining except the area is somewhat wider and certainly less distinct. Normally, the smudged eyelining is continued on the lower lash, too, which creates a fairly intense fringed-lash look, one that is much softer and more natural looking than the firm-edged lining treatment.

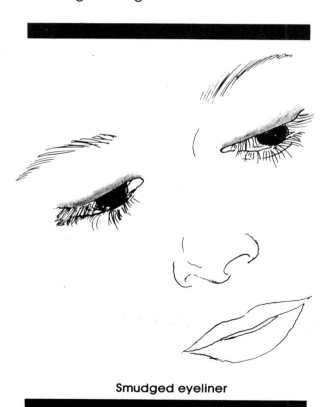

Smudged eyeliner

THE LASHES

The application of mascara is the next step. Mascara creates what is, perhaps, the most dramatic change. By making the lashes look darker, longer, and thicker, mascara defines the eye, makes the whites look whiter, and gives a soft, furry frame.

Some lashes, however, do not have a natural curl. They jut straight out from the lid, shadowing the eye and making it seem smaller. Before any mascara is applied, the lashes should be critically examined to determine whether or not the use of an eyelash curler is indicated. If so, the directions for its use are fairly simple, howbeit delicate.

The lashes are inserted between the scissorlike grips of the curler, with particular care being taken that all the lashes are included. As the handles are tightened, the rubber-protected grips close upon the lashes. While holding the tightened curler for eight to ten seconds, great care should be taken that none of the lashes is pulled or tugged. The handles are released, the curler removed, and the lashes should have a natural looking arc.

If, on the other hand, the lashes form an unnatural looking forty-five-degree angle, wet the lashes to uncurl, and try again, this time tightening the curler upon the lash for less time. You might also like to place the curler on different areas of the lash — at the base or root, then at the middle, and last, at the tip.

Whatever you do, the curling of the lash is not permanent so do not be afraid to experiment until you have complete control and can handle the curler adeptly.

The lashes now being prepared, the application of mascara is next. This step is probably the one which takes the greatest amount of time. It is most important that great care is taken to completely surround each and every lash with the mascara. In this way, each lash will look longer and thicker, and thereby create a lush set of eyelashes.

There are two types of mascara: the cake type and the cream. The first comes in a dry, compressed-cake form. A small amount of water is brushed onto the cake to form a paste, which is then applied to the lashes. The cream type comes in two forms: in a tube, the contents of which is squeezed onto a brush and then applied, or in wand form. The wand type comes complete with its own brush attached. As the brush is removed from the mascara in which it lies, a rubber wiper removes the excess mascara and the application is achieved with the remaining mascara.

The lashes should be deeply embedded within the mascara brush so that they are completely surrounded by the bristles. Each lash is then coated, but you must be careful that the lashes do not form thick clumps but individually swing out from the lid.

For easier non-smear application, the bottom lash should be done first. In this way the wet upper lash is not raised against the brow bone.

Look up into a hand mirror until the lower lashes are as far away from the skin as they possibly can be. Moving the brush sideways, apply the mascara with the point of

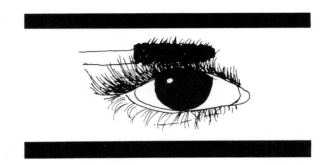

the brush. (Be careful not to poke the eye.) Now, using the side of the brush, arrange the lower lashes into a normal downward sweep. Do both lower lashes.

For the top lashes, lower the hand mirror until the upper lashes are as far away from the brow bone as possible. Continuing to look down into the mirror, apply the mascara, using the side of the brush. Push each lash down into the bristles, dividing and coating each one.

If, regardless of the care you take, smudges and smears do occur, merely disregard them until the complete application has been accomplished. The then-dried mishaps can be easily flicked away with a tissue or Q-Tip.

For added emphasis a double application of mascara may be applied. The important thing is to maintain the individuality of each lash when applying a second coat. This second coat sometimes tends to make the lashes stick together in unattractive clumps. This is to be prevented.

The proper selection of the shade of mascara is important, too. Black mascara on anyone but a dark brunette has a tendency to give a hard look to the face. It is, therefore, recommended that all blondes, redheads, and light-brown-haired women wear brown mascara.

It is also possible to augment the lid-contour-highlight eyeshadow color family by choosing a mascara of that same particular shade. There are blue, green, purple, maroon, and even gray mascaras available. Or you might like to experiment with a two-toned effect. One shade is applied on both upper and lower lashes. When it dries, seconds later, another, lighter color is applied to the tips only.

Now that the mascara has been applied, your next step is to decide whether or not false lashes are necessary. It was mentioned before that mascara is the cosmetic item which, perhaps, makes the most dramatic difference in the way the eye looks. That should be amended to point out that false lashes can be regarded as extra lashes which have been mascara-ed. False lashes can make an incredible improvement. As a matter of fact, many women look as if they have spent a great deal of time on their faces when all they have done is apply false eyelashes.

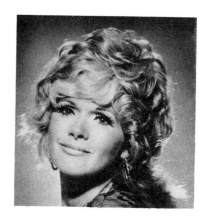

My eyes are my best feature. I prefer powder eyeshadows and my favorite eyelid shade is Dresden blue. I generally use blue as the eye contour color and white for my eye highlight color. (I never try to match my eyeshadow color to my outfit.) I line my eyes, put on two coats of mascara—and sometimes, I wear false eyelashes. I don't highlight my cheekbones, but I contour my face with bronze gel, usually putting it on my forehead, nose, cheek hollows, and chin. And I always wear lipstick—my favorite color is a light beige. I'd be lost without beige lipstick and a smile.

CONNIE STEVENS

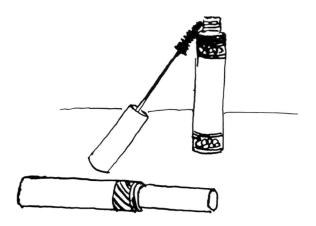

In order for false lashes to look well, the first step is the proper selection. It is important to select the pair that will look less false and more natural. Forgetting, for the time being, stage and other professional occasions when heavy lashes are needed to counteract distance or harsh lighting, the best false lash is that which looks fairly natural when applied.

Many factors contribute to this proper selection: the personality of the wearer, the occasion, the wearer's self-image, and the shape of the eye.

Relative to the eye shape, the lash should be choosen to harmonize, augment, and emphasize the steps already taken to improve or alter the existing shape, size, or structure.

A small, closely set eye would do better with a fine lash that has longer hairs at the outer corner than at the inner corner.

A deeply set eye should wear a fine, even-length lash.

The lash for a drooping or turned-down lid should be similar to that worn on the closely set eye but of more medium thickness.

Basically speaking, however, most women can wear a fine or medium-thick lash which has been feathered to resemble a natural or real lash, i.e., have short and long hairs side by side. It should also be designed to have short hairs at the inner corner and somewhat longer hairs at the outer end.

False lashes come in a wide variety of styles; it would be impossible to describe them all here. When looking at the different styles in a department store or drugstore, simply remember the effect that is desired, remember the means already discussed in attaining this effect, and then choose the lash that would most easily adapt. In many places you can actually try on one of the lashes. This is the ideal situation.

Most lashes are a little too long from corner to corner for the lid. This is purposely done so that you can trim the lash to the exact length needed. Peel the lash from the mount by gently pulling from the outer end. With the adhesive that remains on the lash from the mount, put the lash next to your own. Start at about where your own start and continue to pat the lash into place just above your own. If the false lash extends beyond the outer corner of your eye or where your own lashes end, mark the excess in your mind.

Remove the lash and snip this excess off with a scissors. Always remove the excess from the outer end. It can always be identified as the one with the longer hair. In cases where both ends look identical, it really doesn't matter which end is snipped . . . as long as the snipped end is then considered the outer one.

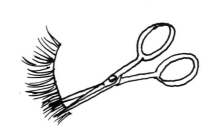

Trimming band of lash

Once the selection has been made, the band should be broken. **Breaking the band** simply means rubbing a fingernail over the band to make it softer. Hold the lash between the thumb and the index finger, the back of the band toward the approaching thumbnail of the other hand. Now, gently rub the nail all along the band. You will notice that as you do this the band forms a more acute horseshoe. The hairs tied onto the band spread and appear more fluttery and feathered.

Normally, a good grade of surgical glue is provided in the box with the lashes. The glue is important. It should dry clear and dry fast. It should also be removed from the lash in one continuous string. If your glue does not measure up to these standards, throw it away. It is either old or of inferior quality. Surgical glue is easily obtained. It appears chalk white when wet but dries perfectly clear.

There are also colored glues on the market. Frankly, they do not perform as well as the clear type and have no real cosmetic value. Rather, they create problems if they are not applied correctly.

Some glues come in tubes, some come in bottles. The latter have wands which are attached to the bottle cap. These are by far the easiest to use. The wand is passed over the band of the lash, and the lash is then ready to be applied. In the case of the tubes, there are two methods of application. A thin line of glue is applied to the band, directly from the tube. If you are able to control the flow of the glue from the tube this is probably much less time-consuming than squeezing a blob of glue out of the tube, inserting a toothpick, and passing this glue-laden toothpick over the band of the lash. Experiment and see which method you prefer.

The most important thing is that you confine the application of the glue to the band **and the band alone**. There is nothing quite so unattractive as a dirty, matted false lash — it is so obviously false.

If you do happen to get some glue on the hairs, be sure to clean it immediately. If the glue will not pull away, clean the entire lash and begin all over again. Glue-laden hairs are impossible to disguise.

The easiest way to apply a false lash is with a tweezer. Grasp the middle of the lash with the tweezer and, looking straight into a mirror, transfer this lash onto your own. Get

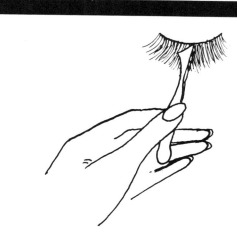

Hold lash with tweezers

the band of the lash as close to the root of your own lashes as possible. There should never be any bare skin exposed. As you push the middle of the lash onto the middle of your lid, the two ends may fly up slightly. Do not let this upset you. One by one, grasp each end with the tweezer and place it correctly. The lash should be affixed to the skin directly above the root of your lashes, not to the lashes themselves.

If any glue smudges onto your skin, simply touch it with your fingertip. It will affix itself to your finger and, in that way, be easily removed. Since it is clear, any slight residue will not show.

Although false lashes are currently out of vogue, do not hesitate to wear them if they enhance your appearance. Keep in mind that the observer should **never** suspect that all those lashes aren't your own. You must exercise the most brutal assessment in honestly evaluating just exactly whom you're fooling!

In the beginning, the use of a three-way mirror is recommended. In this way you can see the lash from all angles. Remember, that's how an observer sees you! Once you get the knack, the application of the lashes shouldn't take you more than a couple of minutes. Although it may be exasperating at first, do not fool yourself into thinking little discrepancies won't matter. They do. As a matter of fact, they give the whole story away and one can hardly strive for a fresh, natural look with lashes zig-zagging up and down on the lid. Take the time to replace them properly.

Sometimes the lash looks fine on the open eye but curls at the base when the eye is closed. Remember that people see you this way, too. You blink, you look downward, etc. Take the extra care that's needed to maintain good grooming, when it comes to the lashes, too.

The use of bottom lashes is yet another way of opening up the eye. It also balances the fringed, furry effect. However, great care should be taken in the application.

After the band has been touched with

glue, the lash is applied most easily by looking upward into a hand mirror. The natural lashes are, in this way, away from the skin. The false lash is applied with a tweezer to the skin directly below the root of the natural lashes. The band of the lash should be pushed up as far as possible into the natural roots so that the false lashes seem to emanate from the natural roots.

Again, place the middle of the lash to the middle of the lower lid, and then affix each corner. Push the hairs of the false lash upward so that they comingle with the natural lashes.

Some women prefer individual lashes or individual clumps of lashes. The latter may be formed by simply snipping a band lash into little clumps. The single, individual lashes are purchased. Frankly speaking, these tiny lashes are best applied by a second person rather than by yourself — that is, unless you have patience, a steady hand, and a three-way mirror. Each hair is picked up by the tweezers, dipped into the special glue, and applied to the **natural lash**, not to the skin.

Individual lashes, properly applied, look lovely and natural. They have the advantage of lasting much longer than the band lash, which is, of course, applied each time. The disadvantage of the individual lashes, however, is that great care must be taken so that they are not bruised and misshapen while sleeping, do not get pulled off while toweling the face dry, etc. In other words, changes in habits such as sleeping, showering, and face cleansing must be made in order to prevent the lashes from being pulled or tugged out. Another disadvantage is that the false hairs have a tendency to pull out the natural lashes.

The special glue that is used to affix the individual lashes is much stronger than surgical glue. It must be removed with a solvent and, in most cases, is a dark brownish black. Do not use this glue for anything other than false individual lashes. Once applied, the individual lashes cannot be reapplied. The residue of glue which clings to each hair is almost impossible to clean off.

The band lash, if treated properly, can last an indeterminable length of time. Proper care involves thorough cleansing after each wearing and storage upon the mount on which they rested when they were purchased. There are cleansers especially prepared for false lashes, or you can use any good eye make-up remover. The type that comes via a saturated pad saves one step.

To clean the lash, it is placed on a firm surface and held steady with one hand while the saturated pad is wiped over the lashes until all the clinging mascara, glue, and dust particles are cleaned away. Then turn the lash over and repeat the process. Blot any excess cleanser from the lash with a clean tissue. Place the lash on the lash mount and close the box to protect the lash from dust. After each wearing, clean the lash by holding it in one hand and, starting at the middle, pulling the glue away.

SHAPING YOUR FACE — THE CHEEKBONES

For many years, a woman's beauty was directly related to how closely her face came to the accepted standards of "perfect proportions." These so-called perfect proportions were a symmetrical arrangement of classic features distributed upon an oval-shaped face.

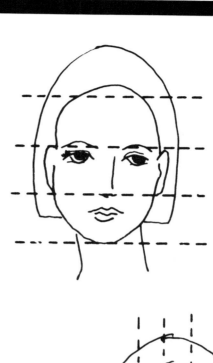

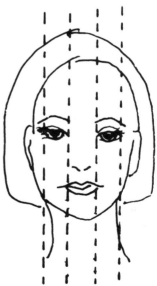

Perfectly proportioned face

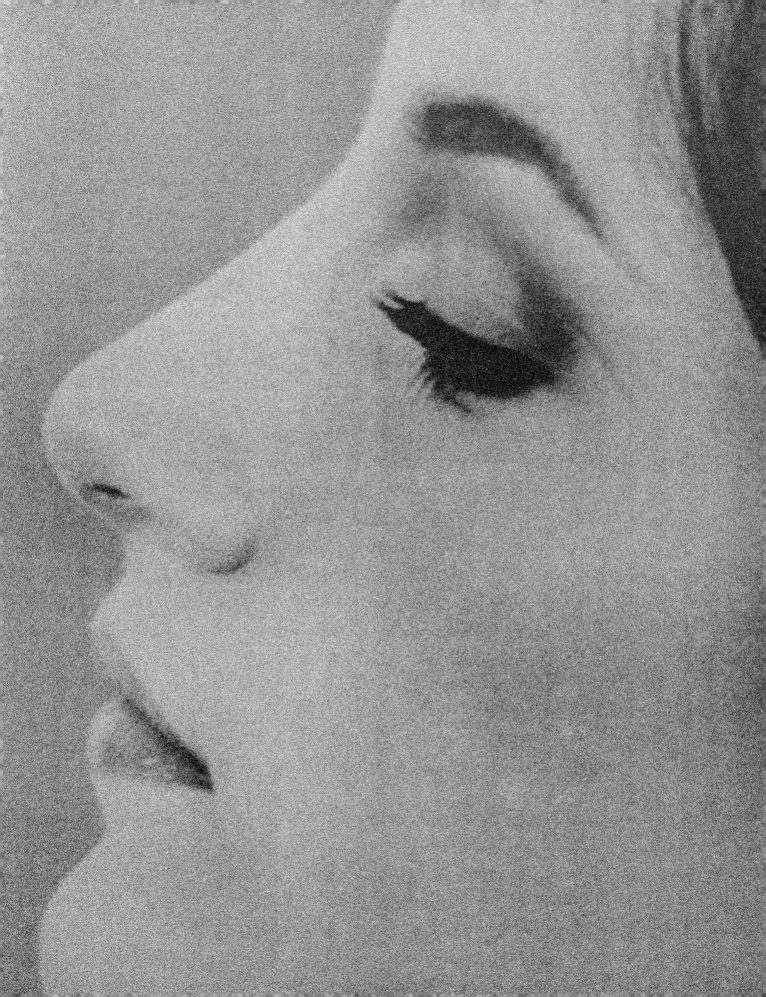

Today's standards of beauty are, happily, much less rigid and much more intelligent. Beauty is no longer the mathematical, slide-rule calculation of A relative to B, juxtapositioned with C. Beauty is the undefinable essense that sets one person apart from another, makes one person attractive to another, and mysteriously rivets attention. Beauty can be only skin deep or it can emanate from within. Beauty is an individual quality.

There are, however, certain elements of the classic acceptance of beauty that must, by necessity, be carried over. These elements are those which hold true not only for beauty of the face but also in the fine-art awareness of beauty of composition, beauty of balance, and beauty of harmonious dimensional planes. All these elements must be considered when approaching the task of making up the face so that its best features are emphasized.

As the skin acts like the artist's canvas, the structure of the cheekbones are the framework over which that canvas is stretched. By and large, the cheekbones affect the overall shape of the face.

There are several distinct face shapes: oval, round, square, triangular, inverted triangle, heart, oblong, and diamond. And there are infinite combinations.

The oval-shaped face is considered to be the most pleasing to the eye, affording the most advantageous background for the balanced and harmonious distribution of features.

That is not to say that all other shapes should be concealed under heavy veils. Indeed, many other shapes make for highly attractive, even **more interesting**, faces. Whether or not to augment this individuality is a question that must be answered by individual tastes. Speaking generally, however, the oval face gives the observing eye a more easily recognizable, more conditioned reflection of accepted beauty standards.

It is sometimes helpful in evaluating what must be done in terms of corrective make-up to define the exact shape of the face. If you cannot clearly see the shape, tie the hair back away from the face. Stand in front of a mirror and draw the shape reflected with a piece of soap. Step back and look at the drawn line. Which shape does it most closely resemble?

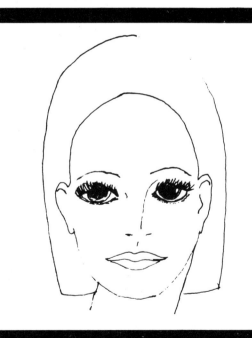

THE OVAL FACE: The temples are the widest part of the face. The jawline is the narrowest.

THE ROUND FACE: The face is widest at the cheekbone, and the face is about as long as it is wide.

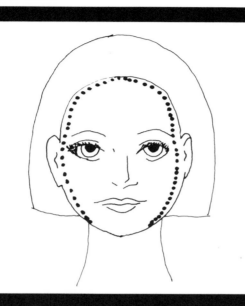

THE SQUARE FACE: The forehead, the temples, the cheekbones, and the jaw all line up to form one straight line down the face.

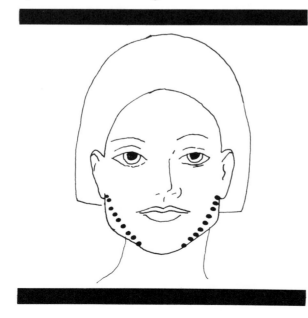

THE TRIANGULAR FACE: The jawline is the widest part of the face. The forehead is much narrower.

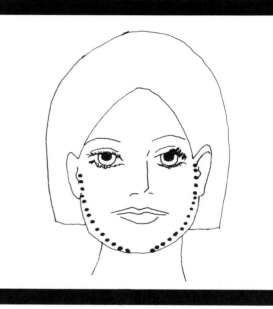

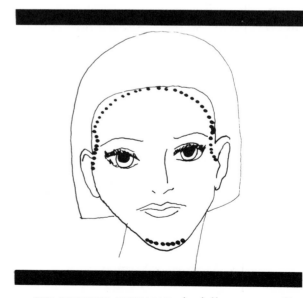

THE INVERTED TRIANGLE: Just the opposite of the triangular, the forehead is the widest part of the face, narrowing down to the chin.

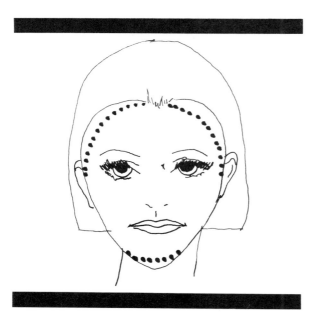

THE HEART FACE: The face is widest at the cheekbones. The forehead is slightly less wide while the jawline and chin are sharply convergent.

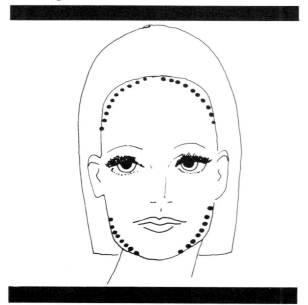

THE OBLONG FACE: This face is closely related to the square face except that the

jawline is slightly rounded down to the chin and the forehead is less broad.

THE DIAMOND FACE: The forehead and the jawline and chin are the narrowest parts of the face; the cheekbones, the widest. Very like the heart-shaped face except that the forehead and jaw are more equal in width.

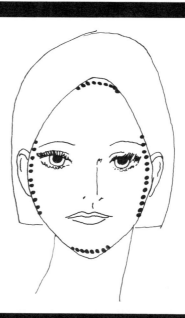

When optically adjusting, softening, emphasizing, or even totally altering the shape of the face, the most crucial step is the application of common sense.

You have already learned that a dark color will absorb the light, making an area recede optically or look much smaller. You have also learned that a light or bright color will reflect the light, making an area seem larger or more prominent. To top it off, you have learned that, used together, the con-

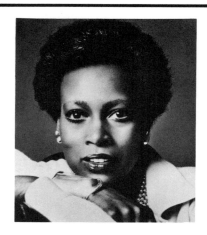

I prefer a liquid foundation, and I always use powder, too. On my cheeks, I use my favorite burgundy powder. On my eyes, I use a charcoal black shadow. My lipstick is a burgundy, plum and cherry mixture. Lipgloss (a must) is my own mixture of my favorite color, burgundy (again). I sometimes highlight my cheekbones with my own mixture, too. When I was a kid, my favorite beauty was Queen Nefertiti. I always contour my own face with a mahogany brown shade. I put it everywhere—on my forehead, nose, cheek hollows, temples, chin, jawline. And then I blend, blend, blend!

NAOMI SIMS

tour color and the highlight color make the effect of each other more dynamic.

Sometime long before the first cosmetic item was applied, the answer to whether or not the shape of the face should be changed should have been answered. This, however, would be the proper time in the make-up application to actually do it.

Changing the shape of the face is accomplished by the means of using the oft-repeated principle of light and dark, or highlighting and contouring. The angular aspects of a square jaw can be softened with contour, the roundness of cheek can be made to look more angular with contour and highlighting. Every conceivable facet of the features may be altered optically!

But first let's define the cosmetics used for structuring.

Face contours are usually a brownish red or deep mauve powder or cream; a shade of foundation one tone darker than that applied to the face; or any cosmetic that achieves a natural-looking, warm shadow.

Face highlighters should be broken down into two categories: cheek highlighters, and skin highlighters. The cheek highlighters are red based, and they come in a wide range of colors from pink to deep mauve. Skin highlighters are normally white or off-white, sometimes with soft, pastel overtones. If a cheek highlighter is viewed as the main facial highlighting medium, the skin highlighter would then be the super-highlighter — the extra boost.

Cheek highlighters are most often called rouge, blush, or gleamers. They come in a wide variety of mediums: cream, gel, liquid, or powder. In all cases, a cheek highlighter should be applied over the foundation and powder.

The cream rouge normally gives vivid color. It is dotted onto the skin and blended out with the fingertips to the desired intensity.

The gel rouge is designed to give sheer color. The effect is that of looking at the skin through a veneer of color. It, too, is dotted onto the skin and blended with the finger-tips. The intensity of the color is limited. The gel gives the freshest, youngest looking blush to the skin.

The liquid rouge normally affords more opaque color but may also be blended out for a more sheer effect. It is applied as above.

The powder rouge is probably the most popular because it lasts the longest. It gives a wide range of intensity depending upon application. It should be applied with a brush rather than a puff.

All of the cheek highlighters are avail-able in both flat tones and in pearlized shades. The latter achieve a somewhat more effectual highlight because of their reflective qualities. However, the flat tones are adequately effective and, of course, may always be made frosted by adding a pearlized medium.

The role of cheek highlighter is twofold. It gives the face color and it emphasizes the cheekbones. The entire face has only three color zones: the eyes, the cheeks, and the lips. The cheeks are the main factor in what may be called the "positive" aspect of the face shape. The "negative" aspect is that of which the observing eye is not actually con-scious.

A moment more should be spent on further clarifying rouge. Rouge comes in

such a plentiful variety of shades that it is sometimes confusing to the novice. It is vital that the principle of light and dark and the effects of contrasting tones be remem-bered. Whereas a mauvy-color rouge may, in some cases, be applied as a highlighter, it does not preclude the possibility that that same color can also be used as a contour. **The important reminder is that whether it is a highlight or a contour depends entirely on the surrounding colors or tones.**

Do not, therefore, be confused by think-ing that because a color is a "rouge color" it must, therefore, of necessity be a highlight-er.

Skin highlighters are the third item in the structuring trio. They come in cream, liq-uid, or powder form and are, basically, highly pearlized. They are either white, off-white, or light beige. (In some cases, the cream used for concealing circles under the eyes may be used when an unfrosted effect is desired.) Their purpose is to add greater definition, to accent, and to dramatize a structural plane by reflecting available light and/or by creating the illu-sion of light. They are the super highlighters. Generally speaking, the trio of the con-tour/highlight/super highlight are used together because, as mentioned before, they make each other more dynamic.

Now that you are familiar with the mediums, it is important that you under-stand another aspect of structuring. Keep in mind that it's the overall shape of the face that is going to be softened or altered. Do not simply see an individual problem and let it go at that. Everything is relative! A wide

71

forehead could not exist without a narrow jaw. You can't have a face that is too long without having a face that is too narrow!

Each individual "flaw" is handled in relation to the rest of the face. Each must be analyzed with the same attention to its counterpart and all with the same attention to light and dark.

For instance, the round face is round because it is either too short or too wide. Follow? If the sides of the face were to be brought in closer to the nose, the face would look thinner, right? Therefore, the sides of the forehead, the temples, the sides of the cheeks, the jaws are all contoured. Special attention is paid to the hollows under the

cheekbones. This alone makes the face look longer and thinner. To augment that effect and heighten the illusion, a cheek highlighter is applied to the cheekbone. This color makes the bones jut out from the face, giving the face a more angular appearance. This counteracts the soft roundness of the natural face shape. Coupled with the shading or contouring, the face shape has been optically altered considerably. But that's not all. Now the super highlighter is applied. A little blended onto the very center of the forehead thins the face by making that center project. A thin, confined line of super highlighter is also applied to the very crest of the cheekbone. This gives the effect of a personal spotlight shining above the head and the bones of the cheek being so prominent that the light cannot get beyond them. The light is, therefore, trapped on the top of the bone.

The observing eye does not analyze what make-up tricks it sees **unless** they are done unnaturally or with a heavy hand. It sees, instead, that which it is accustomed to seeing — the play of light.

The square face is handled in the same way. Wherever an unwanted or harsh plane lies, a contour is applied to soften and minimize it. The angular jaws are contoured to present a more rounded shape. The angles of the forehead are likewise contoured. A cheek highlighter is applied to the cheekbones to accentuate them. The hollows under the cheekbones are contoured, which not only makes the cheeks less flat

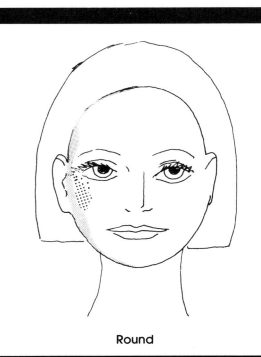

Round

but also gives the cheekbones greater lift and definition. A super highlight is applied along the crest of the cheekbone to dramatize this effect.

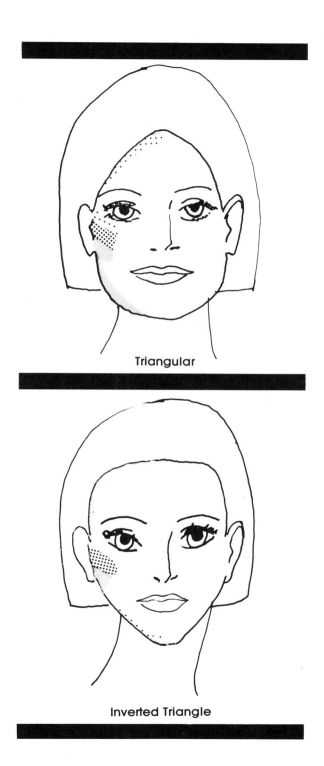

Triangular

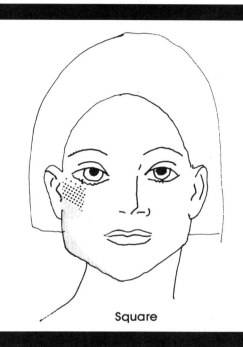

Square

The triangular face is formed by a narrow forehead and a wide jawline. The latter should be contoured, the former highlighted — and then super-highlighted. The cheeks should be defined with cheek highlighter and contouring in the hollows.

The inverted triangle is a very common face shape. The chin is pointed and the forehead is wide. The sides of the forehead down to the temples should be contoured so that the illusion is one of shadow. The converging jawline should be highlighted with a super-highlighter in a thin line along the jaw. The cheek highlighter is applied a little lower than normally and blended down into the super-highlighter. The point of

Inverted Triangle

the chin is softened by the use of a contour, and magnified by a super highlighter in a rounded line above the contour.

The heart face is fairly similar to the diamond or the inverted triangle. Greater balance is provided this type of face by applying contour to the chin, the temples, and the arcs of the forehead. Cheek highlighter is applied to the bone, extending down slightly into the hollows. A super-highlight can be applied above the chin contour and along the jawline.

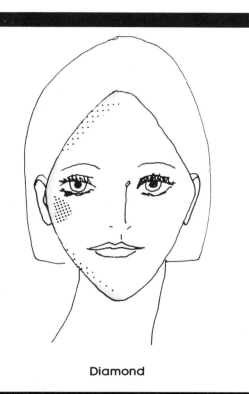

Diamond

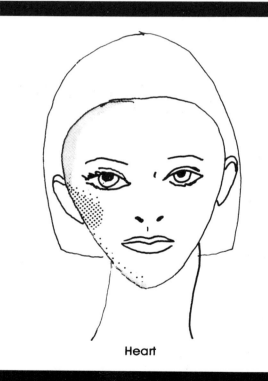

Heart

The diamond is treated as above except the forehead is highlighted with a cheek highlighter all along the hairline. A super-highlighter is then applied in two well blended dots at each side to represent broad bones. The chin is contoured to soften its point and highlighted to a point where the jawline increases in width.

The oblong face is treated exactly like an oval face shape, except that the hairline at the top of the forehead is contoured to make the face look shorter. Cheek highlighter is applied to the cheekbone; super-highlighter is applied above; a scant amount of contour is applied to the temples and directly below the cheek highlighter to emphasize the hollows and exaggerate the cheekbone structure.

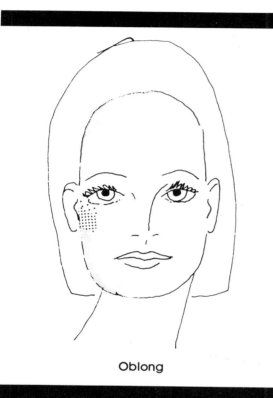

Oblong

The proper application of the highlighting and contouring is, of course, of prime importance in artfully achieving any structuring. If creams are used, they should be dotted onto the area and blended out carefully so as to leave no line of demarcation. If foundation is used for contouring, it too must be blended carefully so that one color tone flows into the other. Powers should be brushed until they are natural-looking rather than obvious. This is more easily accomplished by the use of brushes designed specifically for that purpose. A rouge brush is a rounded, fluffy brush which splays out, giving a soft-looking application. The contour brush, on the other hand, is a flat-tipped brush that gives a more defined application. It should be brushed until all hard edges are blended. The purpose of the flat surface of the brush is to confine the application. It is, therefore, important that you do not use another type of brush unless you want the applied color to cover a wide area.

It is also important that you do not stint when it comes to applicators. **Your make-up is as good as the brushes with which you apply it.** A good brush will last for years and years if it is taken care of properly. For this reason, it is foolish to get low-grade equipment.

As you are contouring and highlighting to change or soften the shape of the face, you may also want to disguise other flaws.

A double chin can be minimized to a great extent by the application of a contour upon the extra layer itself, highlighting the jawline. A weak jawline may be made stronger by applying highlight to the jawline and contouring the area of the neck directly below.

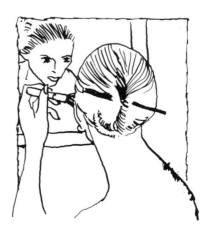

THE NOSE

Probably the most popular corrective make-up tips are those which alter the nose. The nose should be structured (highlighted and contoured) just like every other part of the face. If it is too long, the tip and base of the nostrils are contoured. If it is too wide, the sides are contoured. If it is crooked, the crooked side is contoured, the other side is highlighted, and a straight line of super-highlighter is drawn straight down the nose — disregarding the fact that the line does not equally divide the nose. If it is hooked, the protruding bone is contoured. If the tip is hooked, just the tip is contoured and a dot of super-highlighter is applied. If it is too long and thin, the tip is contoured, and the sides are highlighted. Very often the nose merely requires defining. A contour is applied to the hollows of the nostrils, and a highlighter is placed straight down the nose.

How do you judge if the nose is too long? Basically, the area of the face is broken into three parts. One part is from the hairline down to the bridge of the nose. The second part is from the bridge of the nose (or a line at the level of the brows) down to the nostrils. The last section is from the nostrils down to the chin.

THE LIPS

The lips should lie one-third of the way between the nostrils and the chin, and they should extend to a point just beyond the inside corners of the eyes.

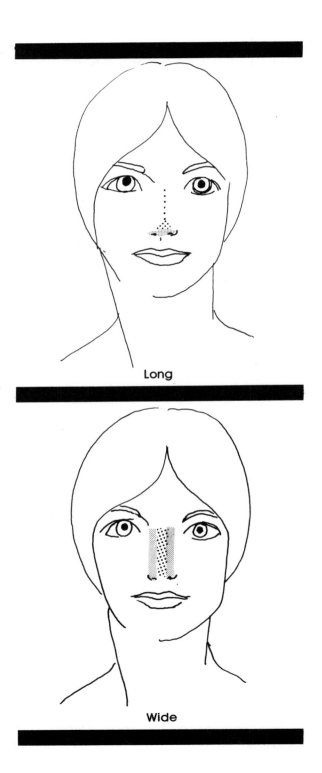

Long

Wide

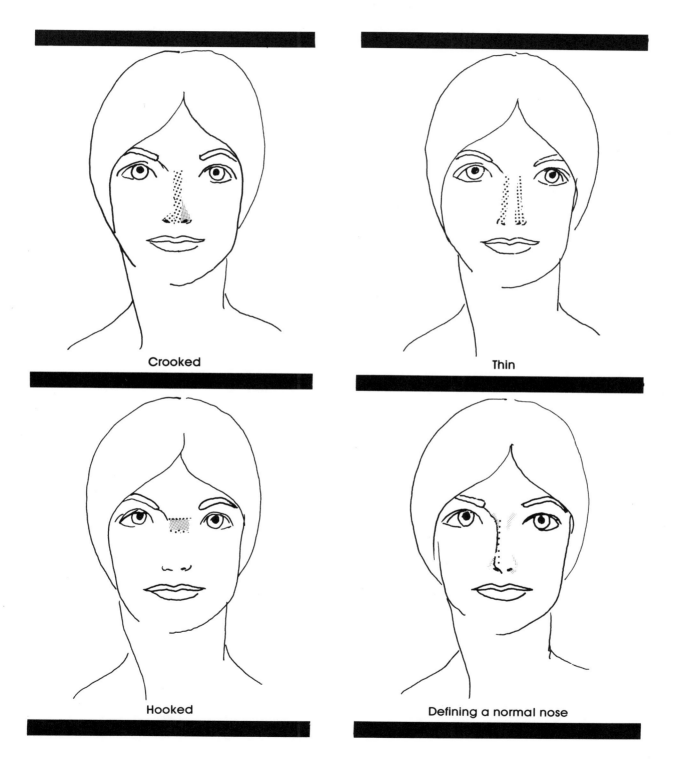

Crooked

Thin

Hooked

Defining a normal nose

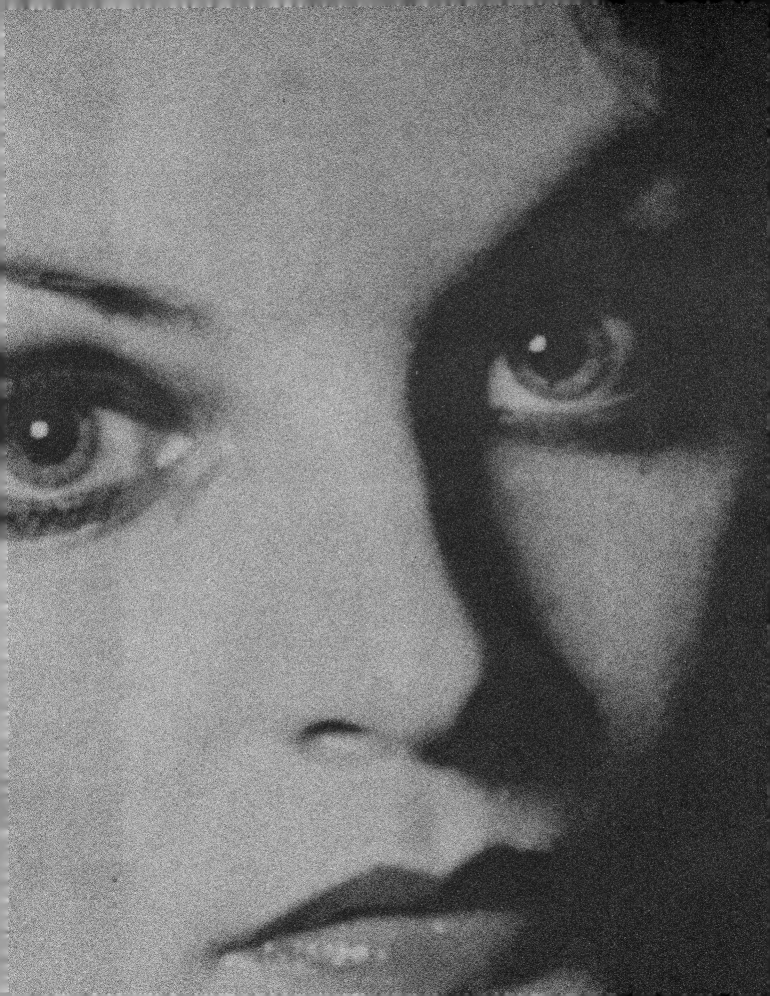

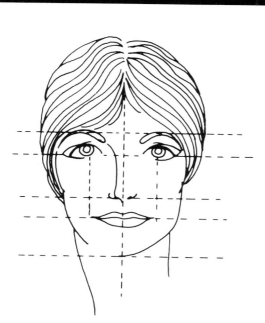

Classically proportioned lips

The application of lip color to the mouth is extremely important. First of all, it makes up the third and last color zone of the face, and second, it balances the face.

The mouth is a very responsive feature of the face. It registers all the emotions and, in most cases, is the feature people look at most when they are not looking "straight into the eyes."

The proper use of color on the lips can affect the whiteness of the eyes, the shade of the iris, and the shade of the complexion. These color variations are all relative to the color wheel, to which colors accentuate and minimize each other, and to the effects of tonal contrasts.

A lip color should be selected, first, to magnify or heighten one's attractiveness. The **second** consideration is the costume. This does not mean, however, that colors that create a dischord should ever be considered. Rather, if the color that looks best clashes with a particular costume, a concession should be made within that same color zone — perhaps a lighter shade of the same color or that same shade blotted down and altered slightly with a tinted gloss. Nor does it mean that there is one color, and one color alone, per person. Of course there are certain shades that look better than others. However, variety is certainly the spice of a woman's life, and she loves the different images she can reflect. The only recommendation is that one should first evaluate the total effect rather than brashly going hog-wild simply because the color, itself, is captivating.

Again, there are no firm rules when it comes to color selection. A guide, a very **vague** guide, for the beginner is that fair-skinned women look best in light tones, dark-skinned women in bright tones, unless the lips are thick. Black women with rather thick lips should wear deep, brownish reds or mauves. The only rule, which is of rather a mild variety, concerns redheads. Because of the shade of their hair, redheads should not wear a lip color that is pale or pink or fuchsia. Redheads look best in true reds, oranges, and in the russet shades. Brunettes and blondes can really wear any color, depending on their overall skin tone.

Experiment with color to see how it affects the skin. See how some clear reds make the skin look whiter, how fuchsia or bluish reds make blue eyes seem bluer, how orange tones make slightly off-white teeth

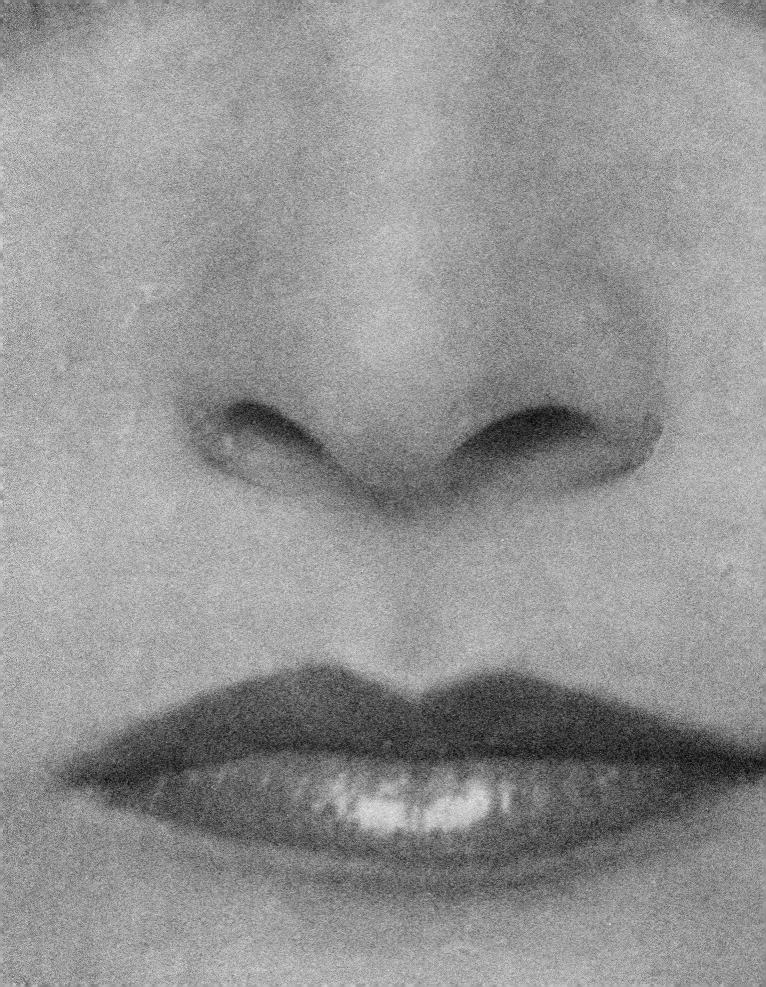

look yellower. All these factors, and more, should be considered when selecting a lip color.

The size and shape of the mouth should also be evaluated. If the lips are too thick, a bright color will only accentuate it. Thin lips look thinner with dark shades. In other words, the same principles of light and dark apply!

The first step in making up the lips is preparing them for the application of lip color by applying a veil of foundation and powder over them. The foundation/powder acts in two ways: It supplies a good base on which to work, giving the lip color greater durability and, second, it gives the lips a softer outline on which to either apply the lip color along its natural edges or to subtly alter that natural outline.

The second step in making up the lips is to outline them. The purpose of this outlining is to give the mouth a crisp, clean shape. As it is impossible to achieve this by using a tube of lipstick or a fingertip, there are two implements recommended: a lipliner pencil, or a lip brush. Of the two, the pencil is probably the easiest to use. They are grease-based and similar to eyebrow pencils. Another variety is the ultrasoft, fat eyeshadow pencils, in an appropriate shade, naturally.

A good brush is one that comes with a cover (to prevent dust and dirt from clinging) and is made of sable. Sable hairs flip right back into position without crushing down. That is why sable makes the best brushes. A lip brush should be fairly firm, so as to execute a crisp line, and should not splay out as does a powder or rouge brush.

Pencils should be kept honed so that the line they draw is thin and hard-edged. Natu-rally, they should not be **so** pointed that they hurt the sensitive lips. Brushes should be carefully wiped after use and thoroughly cleaned before the application of each new color. If this is not done, the color which is transported will not be the true color but a combination of the new with the old. The brush should, of course, be kept clean for hygienic purposes, also.

To outline the lips, keep the mouth in a natural, closed position. Starting at the cupid's bow, draw the two tiny diagonal lines which define it. Now draw a line from the crest of the bow down to the corner of the mouth, on each side. To outline the lower lip, starting at the center, draw a line out to each corner. Open the mouth slightly so that the inside corners are exposed. Draw the outline into these corners.

In the beginning, it is sometimes helpful to dot the lips before actually drawing the line. Dot each cupid's bow crest, the corners and the middle of the lower lip. Now, draw lines from dot to dot.

When using a brush, it is important that you have enough lipcolor on the bristles to execute a crisp line. Stop after each stroke and collect more color.

The shade of the lipliner depends on the shade of lip color. They should blend together so that neither one is individually obvious. When using a brush, this is easy because the outline is made with the same color. When a pencil is used, however, greater care must be taken because pencils do not come in as wide a variety of shades. For that reason, select a shade that will harmonize and blend into the lip color choice.

This is important when it comes to corrective lip color techniques, also. Anything obvious or readily seen cannot be considered effective either in the lipline area or in any other, for that matter.

To optically alter wide, full lips, draw the lip outline just barely within the natural one. The foundation plus powder covering the natural lipline will conceal it to some extent. Use a slightly darker liplining shade and then carefully blend down into the lip color.

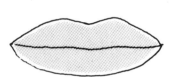

Full

For thin lips, apply the lipline slightly above the natural one. If the existing lipline is sharply defined, use a slightly darker corrective lipline above it. Blend carefully with a bright or light lip color.

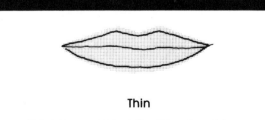

Thin

For unbalanced lips, correct the balance by drawing the lipline along the natural line on one lip and extending the line above the natural line on the thinner lip. Or vice versa. Or use two different shades of lipstick. The lighter shade on the thinner lip, the darker on the other. (These two shades must not be more than two shades apart in tonal quality.)

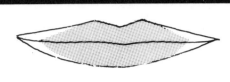

Wide

For nondescript lips, draw the lipline desired using a brownish red or maroon lip color.

If the lips are too wide horizontally, shorten them slightly at the corners.

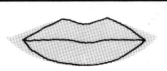

Short

If they are too short horizontally, lengthen them slightly by extending the normal lipline.

Although trends come and go with reference to lip color, its value must be acknowledged. Without lip color the face looks top-heavy, the expression vapid, and the overall make-up unfinished. This is definitely not to say that heavy or bright lip colors **must** be used. The point that should be underlined is that **some** color is necessary.

Standard lip color comes in two varieties: lipstick and lipgloss. Lipstick has more concentrated color than the lipgloss, which is more shiny. Lipgloss may be used alone to achieve a gleaming, transparent color or it may be used in conjunction with a lipstick. Both come in a very wide variety of shades. Either one may be mixed together, lipstick to lipstick, or mixed with one another, lipstick to gloss. In this way the very wide variety of shades becomes infinite.

Less conventional lip colors are cheek gleamers, cheek gels, cream rouges, and bronzers. All of these, too, may be combined so that the range of lip colors never ends.

The intensity of application is another method of increasing the variety. Straight from the tube or tub, blotted, applied sparingly or extravagantly — everything is in the touch. The effect is up to you. Sometimes you might like to use the same cheek color as lip color — or you might like to augment the face with a brighter, duller, deeper, lighter tone. Experiment! Experiment! Experiment!

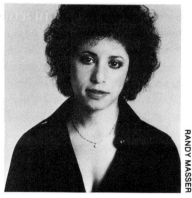

RANDY MASSER

Because my skin has large pores—which I hate—I need to follow a proper diet and get enough exercise. I sometimes give myself facials at home, and when I feel like treating myself, I go for a professional facial. I never use moisturizer. I do use a cream foundation, in a shade that darkens my complexion, and I always wear powder. I like either cream or powder eyeshadows: slate for the eye contour color, blue or gray for the highlight color, and two coats of mascara. When I wear lipstick, my favorite color is a real red, and I add Make-Up Center's Natural Gloss.

JANIS IAN

83

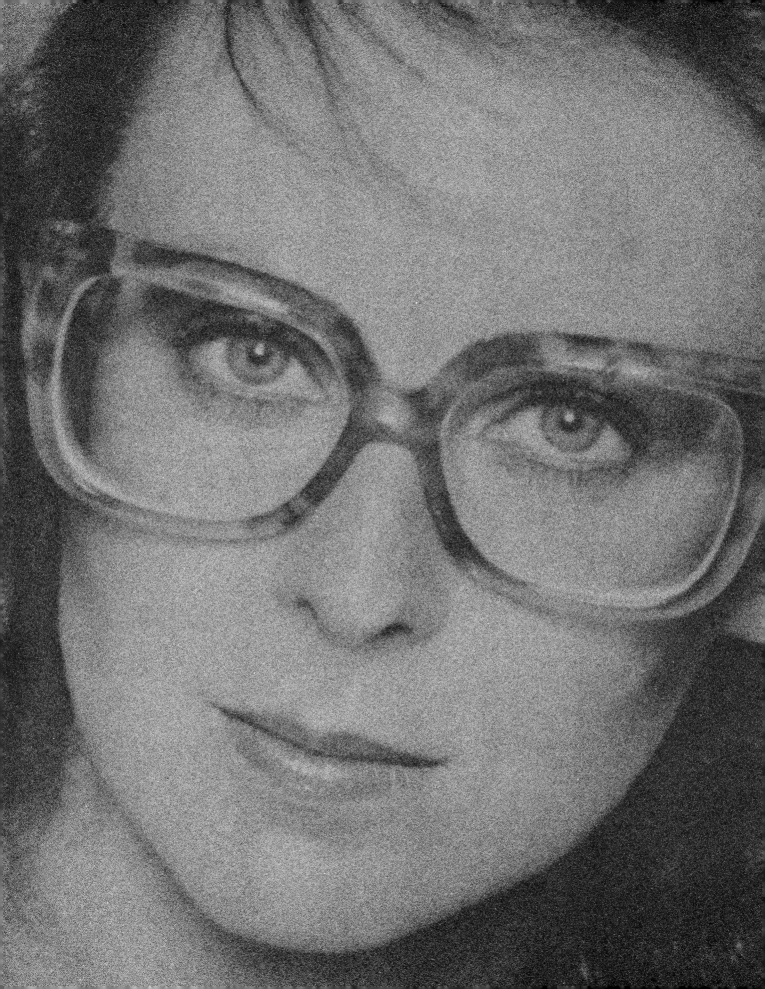

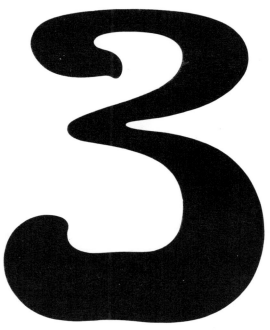

VARIATIONS ON YOUR BASIC MAKE-UP PLAN

EYEGLASSES

Your eyes should look as pretty when wearing glasses as without them! It's all in selecting the correct shape to harmonize with the shape of your face and in the eye make-up that goes on behind those glasses.

It's important to acknowledge that more attention should be paid to the eyes behind glasses. Very often the observer doesn't see past the lens or, in the case of tinted lenses, the total area looks cloudy and nondescript.

When glasses are worn continually, a slightly heavier eye make-up is called for. Another coat of mascara, a slightly more intense application of the eyeshadows, and almost always, a smudge or eye line to augment the fringe of the lash. When glasses are worn intermittently, a compromise between normal and with-glasses eye make-up should be applied. In other words, if the everyday, average eye make-up is applied, it may look fine for those moments when the glasses are not worn but the eyes will look pale and undefined once the glasses are in place.

Before we go into selecting the correct shape of the frames, consider these special tips.

    1. When you try on the glasses, make sure that your eyebrows are either covered by the upper part of the frame or that they are on view

from within. If the brows extend beyond the upper frame it tends to give an unbalanced, quizzical expression.

2. Some large frames, which are now so popular and fashionable, rest on the fleshy part of the cheeks. This may activate the oil glands and could cause blemishes. If you are acne- or pimple-prone, watch out. If you see that you're developing a mild irritation or a series of tiny bumps, try this before you give up: Wipe the base of the frames (the part that rests on your flesh) with a skin toner or witch hazel several times a day. That may control it.

3. If you happen to have a long nose, select a frame with a low slung bridge. The bridge is the part that rests on your nose. It will optically shorten the appearance of the nose.

4. If your nose is broad, pick a dark-toned bridge.

5. If your nose is pinched or narrow or if you have closely set eyes, select a frame which is light-colored.

6. If you have to wear thick lenses, stay away from large frames. The thick lens distorts the entire background and magnifies the pores and lines. If the thickness of the lens creates a bug-eye effect, wear dark eyeshadow to combat the intensification.

7. If you have a big face, regardless of the shape, select big glasses.

8. Don't shop for your glasses when you're in one of your "I'm ugly" moods.

9. Try on a wide variety of glasses before you select one, regardless of what the stylist says or suggests. In the end, it's **you** who has to be happy with the way you look in them, not he or she!

Now to the shapes themselves. For a diamond-shaped face, balance the broadness of the cheeks/temples by draw-

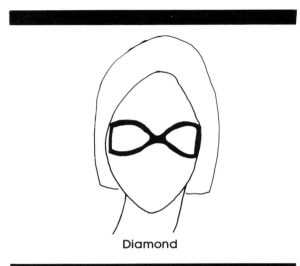

Diamond

ing the observing eye to the forehead or down to the jawline. Therefore, inverted, flared, geometric and round frames are best.

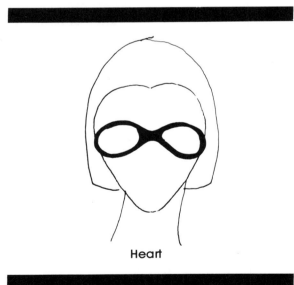

Heart

Heart-shaped faces are best counterbalanced by drawing the eye downward by using a flared geometric or oval frame.

Square-shaped faces benefit from the softening effect of aviators, flared geometrics, rounds, or curved rectangles.

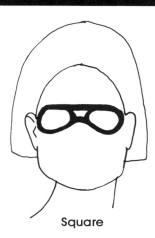

Square

Round faces need greater length. Select a shape that gives that illusion with squares or geometrics.

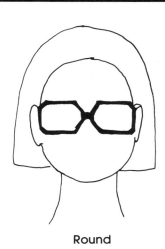

Round

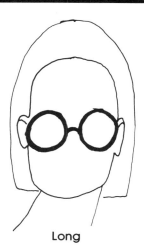

Long

A long face needs more breadth. Emphasize width via wide, deep ovals or rectangles.

CONTACT LENSES vs MAKE-UP

Many people still feel that the use of contact lenses in conjunction with the wearing of eye make-up is dangerous. Their friends tell them so, and even some doctors still recommend doing without. It seems such an anomaly to me. One of the reasons one elects to wear contact lenses, aside from their convenience, etc., is to look better. There's trying to look better on one hand and the exact reverse on the other, the absence of make-up. It just doesn't make any sense!

87

It didn't take too profound a research effort to arrive at the following conclusion. A safe compatability between make-up and contact lenses is available to those who will follow some simple preliminary precautions.

There are two types of lenses, the soft and the hard. Since the soft type can absorb oils and even certain colors, it is recommended that they be inserted before the application of make-up. In this way they are fairly protected unless, of course, make-up is inadvertently and accidently poked into the eye. Before inserting the lenses the hands should be washed with unscented soap and thoroughly dried with a lint-free towel. The hard lenses will not absorb color or oils, but their edges are somewhat thicker and firmer. It is recommended that they be inserted **after** the make-up application, since even the most delicate touch on the closed eyelid can feel uncomfortable and may even dislodge the lens.

Some simple rules to follow for any contact lens wearer are:

1. Be especially careful to tap the end of the brush to dislodge any clinging powder particles before applying powder eyeshadow. Any little grain can cause irritation and/or tearing.

2. After applying the mascara, allow it to dry a moment or two. Then brush the lashes with a clean brush. Any loose mascara bits will be dislodged and brushed away, preventing them from falling into the eyes later on. **Never** wear the lash extender or the lash thickener type of mascara. This variety is made up of little bits of nylon mixed into the normal mascara paste. These little bits are never all securely fastened to the lashes and have a tendency to drop, irritating the eyes.

3. Never use eye make-up remover while the lenses are in place.

4. Once your lenses are inserted, make sure your eyes are closed when applying any aeorosol spray (deodorant, hair spray, even perfume, furniture polish, paint — anything!) and keep them closed until the spray settles.

5. If you apply corrective make-up to the inside rims of the eyes, do so before inserting the lens. The pulling of the lid may dislodge the lens.

6. Do not use soft cotton wads, balls of cotton, or Q-Tips. The lint is somehow attracted to the eye fluid and creates problems. Mohair, angora, or any similar fabric also creates these problems. Use, instead, a sponge or felt-tipped applicator.

7. Use common sense!

THE SEASONS

Like the trees, your appearance normally changes with the seasons. You wear lighter, brighter clothes in the summer, are drawn to warm forest shades in the fall, etc. Unfortunately, many women maintain the same make-up palette from season to season. Their faces look the same whether it be February or October. Aside from how unfashionable it is to do this, the principal crime is one of which no woman should be guilty: boredom.

It's a cruel word but so is the act of boring the observer into a state of blindness. Do I mean real blindness? Of course not. What I'm referring to is the state in which we are

88

subconsciously forced into no longer **see-ing**. It's reflexive: You know something so well you are no longer even aware of it.

That happens with some people. They wear the same face day in, day out. Year in, year out they always look the same. It's boring! Soon nobody pays attention.

Now, understand. I am not saying that, once you find what looks best on you, you should drastically change it just to create a little excitement. No. What I'm saying is that it is important to create, within those optimum perimeters, certain versatilities.

And don't always trust yourself! Very often we fall into cavernous ruts wherein we think any change is a negative one. For instance, you always wear pale pink lipstick. You started sometime in the sixties, and now any deeper shade makes your lips "stand out like a fire engine." To you, yes, maybe. But to the observer, it might just be the balance your face needed. Don't be timid about trying it for a day or two, catching glimpses of yourself in the hall mirror or in shop windows. Listen to the comments your friends make. Do they say you look so rested, or you're looking exceptionally healthy, or whatever? They may not be aware of what change you made — or if there **was** a change. What they're saying is that it's good.

Go to a professional make-up artist. Let an unbiased, trained person see you in his/her own way. Don't limit his/her efforts and put yourself completely in their hands. More often than not a completely new you will emerge. They can see you clinically, without the little cosmetic surgery that you do in your head every time you look in the mirror. And they know what to do about

what they see. If **you** don't like it, try to stay calm. Let it wear for an hour or two and then look again. See how strangers react to you. (You can tell when they think you're attractive or not!) Let your friends or relatives comment and listen closely. Examine what they're saying. Is it negative because they don't want any changes in you, they want you safe and sound in the image they're accustomed to? Is it negative because they're jealous of your new look, or do they **really** not like it? What if **you** love it and they don't? There's an expression which covers that, but it's hardly ladylike.

So, make some changes. In the winter, try the deeper tones. Let your eyes go a little smoky, wear warm, cozy colors. The eyes can carry more color, and a darker lip color will balance it. You can try your normal lipstick with a darker, sheerer lipgloss on top or switch altogether. Don't neglect your cheekbones. Make the colors harmonize so no unbalanced effect is created.

Come the spring, lift your spirits and that of the observer by wearing clearer tones. Not pale ones but clear colors, i.e., pink instead of dusty rose, green instead of khaki. Let your face reflect what's happening out-of-doors, the rebirth. Wear happy colors.

In the summer, when your skin has been carefully, healthfully tanned, wear the sheer tones that allow your healthy glow to shine through. You may only need a little eyeshadow and lipgloss and always mascara, whatever the season! Your natural color may be all that's needed to give the face one even tone and to burnish the cheekbones — or highlight them with gold powders.

The fall, like the winter, is the time for the earth tones again. Let the sight of your face warm the observer — no frosted pastels, no glaring, cold colors. Stick to the colors of the trees, the land, the twilighted sky.

The important thing is to change! It doesn't have to be "a whole bunch" — even a little makes it!

BLACK SKIN

I want to declare myself, right off. I'm appalled, outraged, and disgusted with article after article, famous beauty after famous beauty, and every Tom, Dick and Harry advocating the premise that black skin is different from white skin — or red skin, or yellow skin, for that matter. I'm sick of it!

Skin is skin, whatever its color! Some skin is oily, some skin is dry, some skin is a combination of both, and some skin is normal. Some skin is pale because of its lack of melanin, some skin is dark because of an abundance of melanin. That's it.

To assume, black reader, that because you are black you must have oily skin is to assume that since all horses have brown eyes, you therefore must be a horse! Ridiculous, isn't it.

Go through the same steps as everybody else who is covered with skin to determine its condition. Analyze it. Does it feel taut and stretched, a size too small? Does it always seem shiny and slightly moist? Are there areas where it looks and feels both ways? Then go back to the chapter on skin which you passed by thinking it was not for you.

There are only two real differences between black skin and white skin. Black skin has a tendency to hypopigment, to get lighter or darker in patches, which white skin does not do so readily. Black skin is often unable to stop the healing or scarring process. It overdoes it and creates the overabundance of scar tissue or raised scars that are sometimes seen on black skin. The slightest injury or irritation creates problems for the black skin and its care should, therefore, be particularly gentle. Very good advice, I think, is to stay away from any harsh products. Mild grainy cleansers should be the limit, and even they should be used tenderly.

Never, never consider a chemical peeling or dermabrasion, even if you can find a doctor who will do it for you! This type of facial work alters the pigmentation of the skin. On pale skins it is not so visible, but on black skin it is definitely as plain as night and day! (Don't feel bad, olive-colored "white" skin shouldn't have it done, either.)

What's the definite plus about black skin? One huge recompense is that black skin stays young-looking longer. Another big plus is that black skin can take more sunbaths than white or pale skins, about three times as much. That is **not** to say that pale black skin will not tan; it will. Another plus — black skin is practically immune to skin cancer because of the melanin protection. That is not to say that blacks never develop skin cancer, only that it's rare. If you are a pale black, use a sun screen, too.

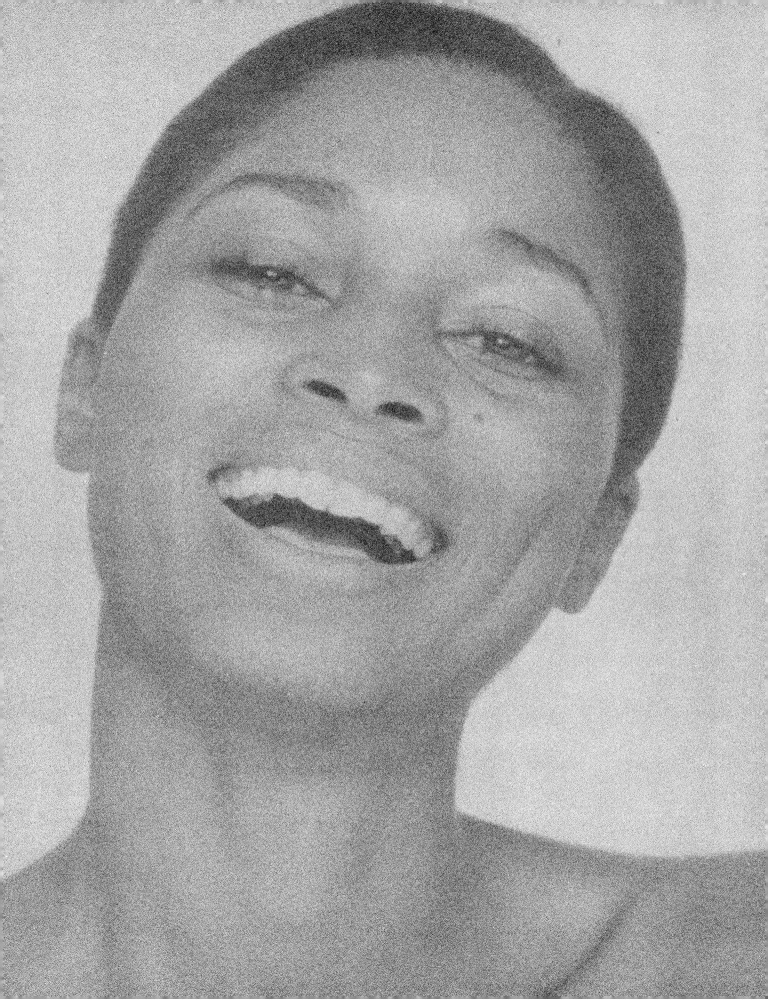

Another plus is the way colors look on your skin. The nonwhite background is the perfect base for those who dislike starkness and bold clarity. Shades that sometimes look too bright or flashy on white skins look wonderful on black. The important thing to remember is that the color you see in the container is **not** the color you get on the face. You must get into the habit of testing **everything**. If you go to a counter that does not have sample displays or products for testing, walk out. (That's good advice for everyone!) And test the product on the area that you intend to put it. Keep in mind that your throat is oftentimes darker than your face, your wrist a different shade than your eyelids. Pay attention to what you're doing to avoid an assortment of expensive, unwearable cosmetics.

And follow the same good skin-care regimens discussed earlier.

PROFESSIONAL MAKE-UP

The term **professional make-up** is usually implemented when speaking of the make-up worn by a professional, a model, an actress, a showgirl, anybody whose income is directly related to the way they look while they are engaged in their work. What is covered in this chapter are the cosmetics applied professionally for professional effects.

Make-up worn during a stage performance, on television, for photographic sessions, for filming, on the runway at a fashion showing, etc., is professional make-up. It's purpose is to beautify, like ordinary street make-up, while also compensating for the wash-out of spotlights, for film idiosyncrasies, or for other inanimate causes that have nothing whatsoever to do with the wearer. By and large, the techniques for applying this type of make-up are the same as for street make-up. The only difference is the amount of coverage and, in certain instances, the placement.

You may wonder why you should bother to know more about this type of make-up since you are not an actress or model. The answer is simple: Because you are interested in making yourself look as beautiful as you can, as constantly as possible.

There are a multitude of occasions when you should alter your make-up application to professional levels. Perhaps you will be called upon to speak at your weekly sales meeting, or you may have volunteered to introduce the guest speaker at the next campaign rally. What about that photograph you've been promising your husband for his desk or that charity convention? These are all instances when your make-up should be altered.

You don't have to be in front of a lot of people and under a lot of lights to look washed out. How about that bank of fluorescents in your office or the daylight streaming onto your face from the window in front of your desk? If you put your make-up on with the incandescent light from your bathroom mirror bulb it will definitely look different when you get under the cold, stark glare of fluorescents, in the gold of real sunlight, or the blue cast by that dismal day.

What it boils down to is this: You don't have to be a professional to need a professional approach to your make-up application. Put your make-up on for the light under which it will be viewed. If you know that the runway at the women's club fashion show is going to be flooded with light, apply enough cosmetics to prevent being washed away by the glare. How much? you ask. It's impossible to describe with words. You simply have to test it for yourself for each and every occasion until you get enough practice to simply know.

Go to the hall and actually see yourself under those lights. It won't take too much experience to note that the pink lipstick that looked so right in the bathroom mirror is now making you look like a ghost. Come to the office early enough one morning to put the proper depth of make-up on to compensate for the lighting, then look at it under normal light levels and try to discern the difference. If it's too drastic a difference apply that which looks good out on the street before you leave the house and then intensify it once you're in the office washroom.

For occasions when you'll be very well lighted with spots, floods, or intensified fluorescents, the guidelines are to contour the cheek hollows to a deeper shadow tone as well as to do any other corrective shadowing. Lipstick should always be brighter than usual; you're fairly safe with a bright true red. Do not be afraid of this color — it's great for street wear, too.

The eyes should be shadowed more dramatically. Use more of the selected shadows and apply them twice as heavily as you normally would. Dark colors always

look brighter; pale colors wash out altogether. Outline the eyes with a finely drawn line or smudge at the mascara line, to accentuate the lashes while defining the eye. Mascara carefully, to thicken the lashes, and refrain from heavy false eyelashes. Aside from looking like heavy false eyelashes, they cast a shadow that is unattractive and disconcerting. Go timidly with highlighters; they reflect twice as much under the glare.

If necessary, buy yourself a floodlight and screw it into a lamp socket that can absorb its wattage. Study your make-up carefully, up close and from afar. Try to see yourself as others will.

For those occasions when you're in shadow — at the commemoration dinner, in the assembly, with the theater group, etc., etc. — just remember that your projection is dimmed. Use brighter, clearer colors. The color brown you usually select for your eyeshadow will look black, the clear blue will look smoky. Compensate for the changes the lighting will make! Your foundation may be a little lighter, the lipstick color a lot clearer, the contouring not as intense as usual. Common sense should solve all the problems.

What about film? That takes in a wide range. There's the local professional photographer and the household candid camera enthusiast, the talk show you may be invited to be on to discuss your new book or your new theory, the convention where your videotaped presentation will be viewed.

Certain basic elements of photographic reproduction must be understood if cosmetic application is to be practiced with any measure of success. Black-and-white film does not see color, it only sees light and dark, plus the whole spectrum of middle grounds. The colors it sees are interpreted as black, white, and shades of gray. Light colors that reflect the light look white; dark or intense colors look black. For example, a pale frosted pink will look white on film and a scarlet red will look dark gray.

This is a very important principle to maintain in terms of black-and-white professional make-up because, obviously, the result of your efforts is only discernible after it has been filmed. A wonderful timesaving device for practicing black-and-white make-up is a videotape machine with which you can immediately see your results. Unfortunately, not too many of us have one available. You **can**, however, go to one of the stores that use this type of equipment in their anti-shoplifting measures. Stand in front of the camera, which is usually up on the wall swinging back and forth across the room. If you're lucky, there'll be a receiver close enough to see yourself. If not, bring a reliable friend to report on how you look. Or go to an electronics store where they sell that type of equipment. They very often have them operating in full view, and you can study yourself close at hand.

In any event, you must select your palette of colors very carefully for black-and-white film. This applies to television as well. Guidelines are as follows. Select the foundation one tone darker to compensate for the wash-out of the lighting. If it's television, you'll have all that bank of lights, and even the snapshot taker has his battery-operated flash. In terms of foundation coverage, unless the skin is perfect, a slightly heavier coverage should be applied to achieve a more matte and even facial tone. Remember, each flaw will cast its own shadow, giving the skin a mottled, uneven texture. A good premise is if a liquid foundation is normally used, select a whipped or creamy one as a substitute.

Special attention should be applied to smoothing this foundation out evenly. You must also be careful to blend it over the jawline so that an unsightly line of demarcation does not exist. You normally do not have to worry about the neck; in most cases it will lie in shadow, anyway, unless special lighting is in effect. If you intend to wear a low-cut gown, blend the foundation all the way down, being careful that the foundation does not soil the garment either in application or in the normal course of sitting or moving the body. The use of a make-up finish spray is recommended after the entire make-up application has been completed. This is a light setting lotion that is sprayed onto the skin with no harmful effects.

Follow up the foundation application with a good brushing of translucent powder to insure a matte finish. What light reflection (or shine) is desired is applied afterward to those areas that will heighten the good bone structure of the face. The powder also helps to minimize the signs of perspiration caused by the heat of the many lights.

The eyes are treated somewhat differently for film than for street make-up. Rather than assessing the shades of color that will augment the iris, the eyes are studied for their shape and dimension. Since the film sees no color, a healthy respect must be paid to the effects of light and dark. The film will see the eyes in shadow, save for a glimmer of reflected light on the lids, if the lids are, in fact, large enough to catch the light. Because the eye sits in a recessed socket that will be interpreted as being even deeper on black-and-white film, an effort is made to bring the eye out toward the viewer.

Light, frosted colors or tints are suggested for use on the lids. Pale pinks, yellows, off-whites, sheerest blues or violets. These colors will project the lid area so that it will appear larger on the film. If the lids are large to begin with, you might try a shade of color that will appear a bit grayer on the film.

The area normally covered with the eye contour color may be augmented by a little touch of contour or not, as you like. A heavy hand, however, is unnecessary. Highlight the area under the brow, as usual, but do not overpower the eye by using too frosted an eyeshadow. Remember that the lights will reflect upon those specks of iridescence, which will look twice as bright.

In terms of corrective eye make-up, the same principles hold as for normal street make-up. When the fold is to be raised, the natural fold is brushed with a light-reflective eyeshadow or highlighter and the man-made fold is created by shading with a contour color. This contour color in black-and-white film could be any color that is deeper than the surrounding colors. However, no one wants to look bizarre, even to those who are doing the filming. Therefore, colors are selected to look fairly attractive in the flesh as well as on film.

The use of an eyeliner is a good medium for further defining the eyes for black-and-white film. It is a **must** for any corrective work, but it also adds depth and clarity to those eyes that normally would not require it.

Mascara should be used on both top and bottom lashes, just as for regular wear. False lashes are also recommended for added emphasis. The length of the lashes should not, however, be so extreme that they cast unattractive shadows. The television camera can be construed as a somewhat dull magnifying glass, the still camera as a somewhat clearer one.

Cheek contour and highlight is very delicate on black-and-white film. Because the film will see a normal cheek color as a shadow, the use of a highlight is recommended for the crest of the cheekbone and should also be blended slightly downward, into the area normally covered by the cheek color.

If hollows in the cheeks are, in fact, present, only a small amount of contouring is necessary; the film will pick up the shadow. Added contour can be made with the normal cheek color or with the normal cheek contour, the latter very delicately. If the hollows do not exist, the corrective technique is to create them with the same delicate approach.

The shade selected for the lips has nothing whatsoever to do with that which should be selected for street wear. Remember it's the **tone** that is reproduced, not the color. Both corrective measures and simple lip application are made with a medium-toned outline and a light fill-in. In every case, the use of a highly pearlized light to medium lipgloss or lipstick is recommended. Although the subject may look slightly washed out in person, the film will pick up the reflections and interpret the tone successfully.

Careful attention can and should be paid to certain lines of the face, too. Normal wrinkles or lines can be minimized by the use of a highlighter. While this technique is incorporated before the application of a foundation in normal street make-up, it is much more effective if applied over the foundation for black-and-white film.

The highlighter or undereye concealer is applied to each and every line with a fine eyelining brush. The smallest, finest brush made is a #00, which is recommended for this delicate work. Great care must be taken to apply this cosmetic to the line itself and not to the surrounding puff of skin.

The correction of an overall face shape is somewhat easier for black-and-white film than it is for normal street wear. Because the film sees tones, and tones alone, changing the structure of the face is easily done with either a deeper shade of foundation or with the cheek contour. The film will see the shadows and translate them to the viewer as either smaller or recessed areas.

MAKE-UP FOR COLOR FILM OR COLOR TELEVISION

The obvious difference between black-and-white film and color film is that the latter sees color. The 35mm film absorbs reds while 16mm, color video tape, and color television exaggerate reds. Therefore, you must allow for these idiosyncrasies when applying make-up for these mediums.

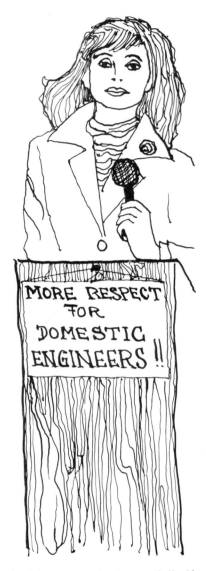

Study this somewhat carefully if you are called upon to be filmed for television, either on tape or live. The normal blues or violets, pinks and oranges, clear reds and russets of street wear must be critically analyzed to determine how the film will affect them. A purple, for instance, is made up of both blue and red. On the normal film your boyfriend or husband bought to take on that trip, you'll look like you're wearing more of a blue violet than a true purple. On television, it may look more like garnet!

The application of the shades and the different cosmetic items is identical to street wear except that a little heavier coverage is called for to compensate for the floodlights.

If you're called upon to model in a fashion show, just intensify. The glare of the lights usually found along the runway makes everything pale. Darken and intensify.

If you're in the local drama group and you're asked to perform, consider the lighting and the size of the theater or auditorium before you make up. The size of a theater is important because of the limitations of projection. Obviously, a person in the first row will see greater detail than a person in the balcony. That person in the balcony, however, should not be neglected. He should see enough to satisfy his eye. Make-up, therefore, is applied so that that balcony audience sees the details of the face. In short, what this means is a heavier application with the use of brighter or more vivid colors.

Another aspect of stage lighting is the gels that are sometimes used over the light fixture. These gels come in a wide spectrum of colors and add dramatization or emphasis. Make-up, however, must be selected in relation to these gels. If an orange gel is used, for instance, the face will look ruddy and all the selected colors will be transposed to a mixture of their original shade plus the orange gel. Blue gels will make the skin look pale and ghoulish, etc.

Great care must be taken in estimating exactly how much make-up should be applied. Efforts should be made to maintain as natural a look as possible, that is to say, to minimize the audience's consciousness of the make-up itself and rightfully focus it on the player.

THE OVER-FIFTY, UNDER-FOURTEEN CROWD

There really isn't enough to say about these age groups to make a respectable chapter, but it is important to say these few things.

Regardless of her actual chronological age, a lady should try to look as attractive and feminine as possible. And when I say "a lady," I'm not limiting it to the over-fifty group! The major part of that effort should certainly be directed to good skin care with somewhat less energy directed to make-up.

Obviously, the girl of ten does not need a cosmetic regimen but she certainly should already be firmly entrenched in the same good cleansing programs as her older sisters. Good skin care should start **early** in order to prevent, as much as possible, the havoc of puberty's skin problems. I think that one of the greatest gifts a mother can offer her children (aside from the usual attributes so well listed in the Scout Oath) is a really good skin-treatment program. Too often parents think that the amount of energy expended in trying to teach youngsters the importance of really cleaning the face just isn't worth the bother. I strongly disagree!

Now, don't get me wrong! I'm not advocating generating a phobia or a psychosis over it — just simple, elementary twice-a-day cleansing, with extras in between for after mud-pie and football sessions. What it does is start a good habit which will last a lifetime. I don't know about you, but it's been my experience that it's much easier to teach them while they're young than to try when they think they know more than you do (about everything!).

When it comes to moisturizing, look at the youngster's skin. It could be dry, too. Let that child begin to apply a little cream at bedtime, or she'll be a ripe candidate for those early laugh lines.

What about the skin of the boy or girl just beginning to pimple? If the aforementioned skin-care techniques have been followed, their troubles should be minimized. If not, it's time to see a good dermatologist, grin and bear it, and know that, normally, it doesn't go on forever.

Young boys should certainly be instructed in the same good cleansing techniques as girls. There is nothing sissy about the trauma young boys undergo during their pimple stage. How much kinder to the psyche if that stage is minimized, **even a little**!

Thankfully, by the time you reach fifty, your pimples are long gone — or should be. What does the mature woman (or man? do to ward off more wrinkling? Basically, nothing can combat the pull of gravity and nothing can **prevent** the signs of age. Maintaining as much moisture within the skin as possible, staying out of the sun, and living in humidified rooms is about all we can do.

What we **can** do is age gracefully and beautifully. There is a rare beauty in a lined face that proudly demonstrates, for all to see, that here is a face that lived life — enjoyed it, suffered from it, was amused with it. Don't hide that beauty via the unobtainable goal of cosmetically masking maturity. It's impossible and looks ludicrous, only highlighting the fact of the age itself and screening the attractiveness that is underlying.

A light, discerning touch is necessary for the mature woman. The same foundation techniques, the same contouring and highlighting, but with the feather-touch of restraint. Colors should be muted, soft, and matte, since high luster only magnifies lined or crepey skin. Bright, bold colors should be avoided on the eyes although a touch of bright red on the lips and cheeks adds sparkle, when applied delicately. If you were always the type of woman to whom the adjectives **dramatic, exotic, singular, bold** were applied, by all means continue your drama and excitement. If, however, you just begin to look "dramatic or exotic" in your fifties, the attempt is often interpreted as "trying to look young" and rarely works.

And what's wrong with getting old, anyway? Certainly it signals the beginning of the end, but look at all the benefits it brings with it. No more worrying about whether or not your girl friend likes you as much as she likes someone else, no more wondering if your braces are really worth the agony they put you through, no more anxiety about whether or not your face will clear up for the school dance, no fretting about sorority initiations, about what major to take. No more fear about never finding Mr. Right, or whether you can really afford to have the baby, or the terrible strain of bringing him up the right way. No more pretending to enjoy the PTA. No more distress at not being able to afford that Ivy League college or disliking your son's fiancée. No more hassle about saying, "No!" when they ask you to babysit for the entire summer or expect you to help buy the new house.

Just the self-fulfillment that comes from knowing you did it all, already, and God willing, you did it well.

So, relax. This is the beginning of the best time of your life.

KITCHEN COSMETICS

There is a great source of beauty treatments right in your own pantry and refrigerator. Some women relish the idea of stirring up a home brew, storing bits and pieces of this and that or even shopping specifically for items to use in their home labs. Other women, by contrast, just can't be bothered. Who's right? Who knows.

I am not a chemist, so I cannot give you **the** definitive answer. My own reaction to kitchen cosmetics is that if it's fun and makes you feel good and if you can see some iota of difference before and after — go ahead. My mother used to say, "It's generally better if you let a professional do it," and I have to agree (or maybe I'm brainwashed!) My educated rationale is that millions of dollars wouldn't be spent every year to let highly skilled scientists **potchka** in expensive

laboratories if the white of an egg could do the same thing as the formulas they spend years developing. I mean, **that** would be some colossal hoax!

Nevertheless, I have collected these recipes from aunts, grandmothers, health nuts, magazines, etc., for those of you who like to fool around and do it yourself. I'm not sure just how much they actually do. I **am** sure they won't harm you!

Keep one very important thing in mind: If the ingredients need refrigeration before your manipulations, they'll need it afterward, too. Make just enough for one application, or store it in the refrigerator. If you do store it, make sure it reaches room temperature before you apply it to the skin, unless it is a toner or eye relaxer.

While we're on the subject, I would like to point out that there are a number of cosmetics on the market which are labeled 100 percent pure, organic, or natural. Look again at the list of ingredients on these products. How long can a totally organic product remain pure and unpolluted without preservatives or refrigeration? When you answer that one, you'll know how 100 percent **pure, organic,** or **natural** that product is.

CORN MILK FACIAL: Grate an ear of corn, gather the mash into a piece of cheesecloth or gauze and squeeze into a clean container. Apply this milk to the face and neck. As it dries, add another layer of the milk and gently massage it in. You can either lie down and enjoy this facial or go about your normal household routine. After about twenty minutes of repeated applications, allow the last layer to dry completely. Then rinse with warm water (do not use soap or cleanser).

It is claimed that, if you repeat this daily for a week or two, your skin should be much improved, with a noticeable difference in terms of skin softness.

CORN MOISTURE CREAM: A teaspoon of corn milk (see above) blended with a dab of sweet butter will, supposedly, produce a dewy complexion out of parchment-dry skin. Let the skin absorb or, when time is brief, rinse off with warm water. (See varieties of sweet butter moisturizers below.)

CUCUMBER MOISTURE CREAM: Add the juice of a crushed and strained cucumber to a dab of sweet butter.

FRUIT MOISTURE CREAM: Add the juice from a freshly pulped fruit to a dab of sweet butter.

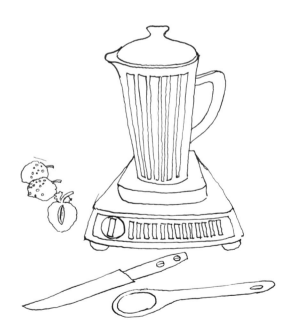

HONEYDEW MOISTURE CREAM: Equal parts of honeydew juice and sweet butter are said to fight fine-line wrinkling. Massage well into skin and leave on for as long as possible.

HONEYDEW ASTRINGENT: A lotion of honeydew and spearmint leaves or any mint leaves makes a deliciously scented toner. Drop half a handful of mint leaves into the blender along with two tablespoons of honeydew melon. Blend very briefly and apply. Rinse with warm water. Or strain through gauze and massage into skin. Do not wash away.

MINT BATH: Mint makes a savory lotion, one especially good for oily skin. It can be applied warm (to open the pores) or cold. A handful of leaves in a cup of water makes a fine brew.

PEACH MOISTURE BOOST: Drop half a freshly skinned peach into the blender with one-fourth teaspoon each of apple cider vinegar and honey. Blend it into a paste. Pour into clean container, adding the contents of a vitamin A and D capsule from fish-oil sources. Rub the paste into the skin and leave on for thirty minutes. Rinse off with warm water. If the vitamin scent lingers, rinse the face with a mint bath.

PEACHES AND CREAM MASK: Equal parts of freshly pulped peaches and cream, apply to the face and neck, let dry and rinse with warm water.

TOMATO CLAY PACK: Mash together the pulp of one tomato and enough fuller's earth (available at most health food stores or pharmacies) to make a smooth paste.

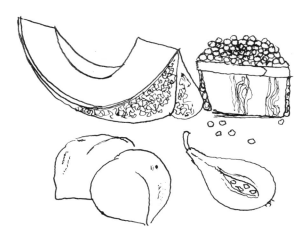

Apply to the face, avoiding the areas around the eyes. Allow to dry and then rinse off with warm water. The tomato is an astringent medium, the earth the blotter which absorbs excess oil from the skin.

SEED SCRUB: This facial is purported to be the finest for maintaining clear, smooth, and delicately tinted skin. Seeds from any melon, or a mixture of squash, watermelon, pumpkin, and cucumber seeds ground fine and mixed with milk. Apply to the face and allow to dry; rinse off with warm water.

UNDER EYE SMOOTHER: Cut a fresh fig in half. Apply each half to the area directly under the eyes. Allow to remain at least twenty minutes.

ALTERNATE UNDER EYE SMOOTHER: Odorless castor oil smooths out dry, parched-looking wrinkles. Alternate: Apply the contents of a vitamin E capsule to this tender area.

SALT SHAKER: To cleanse engorged, distended pores, mix buttermilk and salt into a paste. Massage onto skin, rinse away with warm water.

CORNMEAL/EGG MASK: Mix cornmeal with a whipped whole egg. Massage onto face and allow to set for ten minutes. Rinse off with warm water.

PAPAYA PEEL: Mash the pulp of a fresh papaya and apply to the face. The papaya contains an enzyme that removes dead skin cells. Allow it to remain on the face for at least twenty minutes. Rinse away with warm water.

SKIN SOOTHER: Apply camomile tea to the face by drenching a cotton wad, espressing all the liquid to the point where it no longer runs. Allow to remain upon the face for twenty minutes. Especially relaxing for irritated skins. Variation: use skim milk and allow to dry and remain upon the skin.

SKIN BLEACHER: For sallow or ruddy skins, try this bleacher. Apply an even film of milk of magnesia. Allow to dry and continue to wear for about twenty minutes. Rinse off. Variation: Buttermilk or natural yogurt.

CLEOPATRA'S TIGHTENING MASK: Beat one whole egg, one tablespoon of milk, and one teaspoon of honey. Apply to the face and allow to harden. Let remain for as long as possible. Rinse off with warm water.

GRAPE SOFTENER: To cleanse and soften the skin, one source raved about is grapes. Remove the skins and mash the grapes in the blender. Strain through a gauze and rub the concentrated juice onto your face. Reapply as each layer dries until the juice is consumed. Wash off with warm water.

DRY SHAMPOO: Cornmeal, talc, and ground orris root powder are all cleansing agents for dry shampoos. Brush or rub into the hair and then vigorously brush away.

BRAN MASK: Mix a paste of two tablespoons of natural bran, one tablespoon of baking soda, and enough water to soften. Leave upon the face for ten to fifteen minutes, rinse with apple cider vinegar diluted with equal parts of water.

HONEY AND WHEAT GERM PURIFIER: For a mask that has great pulling power for the removal of blackheads, mildly heat enough honey to cover the face, add a tablespoon of wheat germ and mix. Apply to face and let rest for ten minutes. Wash away with warm water.

BLACKHEAD URGER: Make a paste of oatmeal, honey, and the white of an egg. Massage it onto your face for five to ten minutes. Wash off with warm water.

ANOTHER BLACKHEAD URGER: Mix almond paste and water to paste consistency, massage onto face, allow to dry. Rinse off with warm water.

EYE SOOTHER: Warm rosehip tea bags in a cup of hot water. Squeeze to prevent run-

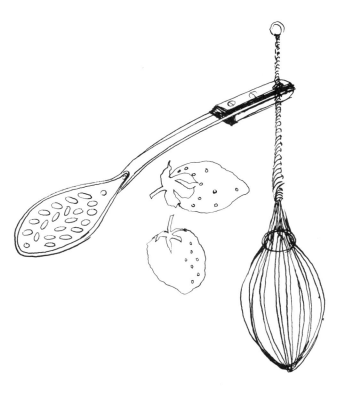

ning water. Apply to closed eyelids. Use the liquid in the cup as a skin wash. Variation: camomile.

POTATO EYE SOOTHER: Grate one medium sized potato. Squeeze the pulp to prevent excess dripping. Apply to closed eyelids.

WRINKLE EASER: Dissolve lecithin granules in warm water and add to vegetable oil, preferably safflower. Apply generously to skin and allow to absorb. This is a slow-acting moisturizer but it, theoretically, works. The combo acts as an antioxidant, while also providing protein.

SKIN TIGHTENER: Apply the white of an egg to the skin. Allow to dry and rinse off with warm water. Or allow to remain all night. This mask temporarily removes wrinkles. Variation: Beat together one egg white, one teaspoon of spirits of camphor, one heaping tablespoon of skim milk powder and a drop or two of mint or rosewater. First apply a film of oderless castor oil to your skin and then follow with a thick layer of this mask. Allow to remain for twenty minutes, then rinse off with warm water.

OILY SKIN LOTION: Equal parts of cucumber juice and distilled witch hazel plus one-half the amount of rosewater. Apply to clean skin. Do not rinse.

PROBLEM-SKIN MASK: Mix four tablespoons of brewer's yeast with enough water to form a dough. Apply to face and allow to stand for thirty minutes.

DRY SKIN NOURISHER: Put half a handful of dried apricots into enough water to cover. Let soak for at least two hours. Mix into a pulp and add enough honey to bind. Apply to face and neck and allow to stand for at least twenty minutes. Rinse off. Apricots are rich in vitamin A, and a vitamin A deficiency can cause dry skin. Variation: Mash a banana, add a drop of honey to bind and apply. Or apply mayonnaise straight from the jar, let stand for fifteen minutes and wash away.

WRINKLE FIGHTER: Beat an egg yoke until fluffy, add a tablespoon of olive oil, and apply to the face. Let stand for fifteen minutes and rinse away. Variation: Replace the olive oil with two capsules of lecithin.

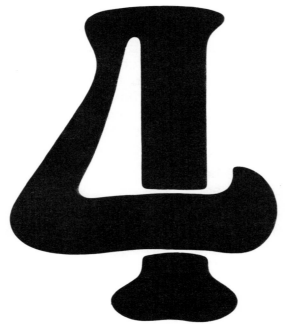

MAKE-OVERS

Make-overs show dramatically what make-up, applied correctly, can achieve in the way of enhancing the appearance. A lot can be learned from make-overs if you carefully examine each individual step.

The purpose of this book is to enable you to do your own make-over (or someone else's). I want you to understand the principles behind what I'm suggesting so that you can apply them to any problem. Remember the one constant, never-changing axiom: Practice and experiment. Don't get discouraged or disheartened if your first efforts don't pay off. Just keep trying; you'll soon see that the image reflected in your mirror keeps looking better and better!

If, however, you do get into one of those slumps (you know the ones I mean . . . you feel ugly and are sure you **are** ugly), then perk up your spirits with a visit to a professional make-up artist. You can usually find one in well-equipped hairdressing salons, big department stores, or cosmetic shops like The Make-Up Center.

Prices for this type of service vary; the range is anywhere from $10 to $150. **Don't be influenced by high prices.** Just because someone charges $100 doesn't necessarily mean that he or she is worth it! Check out their work . . . look at people who leave after an application and see if you like the technique . . . then make your own appointment. Try several make-up artists—it's interesting to see how each one "sees" you. But don't feel that their word is LAW. Take from them whatever you can and wash away the rest!

It's one thing if you're just having a free, fast little demonstration at the counter because you were nabbed on your way to the White Sale, but quite another if what you're buying is supposed to be a lesson/application. Insist that you get your money's worth. Make sure the make-up artist explains specifically what he or she is doing, and why. Don't be embarrassed to ask questions—it's your lesson, you're buying the time! And don't feel that you **have** to buy whatever make-up is suggested, either. Most reputable establishments don't pressure you to buy. (If their product is good, they shouldn't have to!)

If, after one of these sessions, you forget how to do something the make-up artist did, don't feel reluctant to go back and ask. A reputable shop will be glad to explain it over again. Most places offer you a little chart to help you remember where to put what color and what applicators to use. If a chart is not provided, take notes yourself. And remember, don't be two-faced! Don't have one face for special occasions (via a session with a professional) and another for everyday.

You have this book in your hands right now, so use it! I can't tell you how really simple it is to make yourself look absolutely smashing once you get the hang of it . . . and the best part is that you don't even have to start out pretty!

If you need any further encouragement, just picture yourself in a Paris cafe with someone who looks like Humphrey Bogart lifting his glass to you and saying, "Here's looking at you, kid!"

BETTE

Bette is a natural beauty whose features only need clarification. Having good, even-toned skin, Bette needed only a sheer film of liquid foundation and a dusting of translucent powder. Her brows were extended to frame her eyes better. A taupe powder shadow was brushed on, and then fine hair-like lines were drawn in with both ash and light brown pencils to represent Bette's own two-toned brows. The somewhat puffy area under the brows was optically lifted by shading with a loden green cream eyeshadow. Pale yellow cream was applied above the contour to give even more lift, and a powdered gold was applied to the lid. A smudgeline of charcoal brown eyeshadow pencil on both upper and lower lids defined the shape of the eye, and mascara added the finishing touches.

Bette's nose was shortened by a touch of contour powder at the very bottom, between the nostrils. The creases of the nostrils along the sides of the nose were contoured to make the nose look more chiseled. The flare of the nostrils and the tip of the nose were then touched with a cream highlighter for additional definition.

The lines from the nose to the lips were minimized by applying an undereye cover beneath the foundation. Cheek contouring created hollows under the cheekbones and Bette's cheekbones were further emphasized by applying an orangey pearlized cream and highlighting it with a dust of gold along the crest.

Her lips were balanced and defined with a light brown pencil and filled in with an earth-toned gloss. To create the impression of finely chiseled face, a cleft in the chin was added by applying a touch of contouring, and touches of liquid highlighter on what would be the high points of a natural cleft.

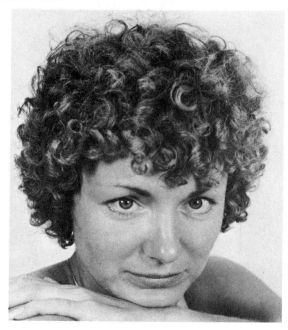

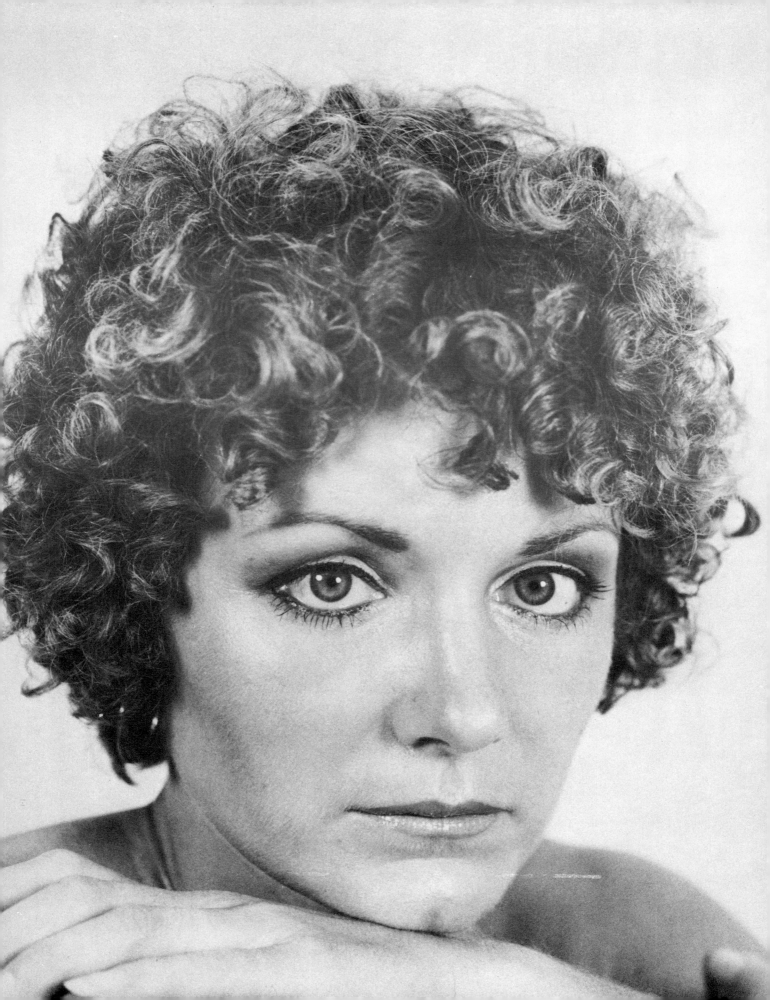

KANDICE

Kandice is a beautiful girl who needs very little help to bring her natural good looks into focus. First, a liquid foundation and powder were carefully applied. Her distinctive eyes were extended at the ends by first laying down a background of taupe-colored powder shadow and then drawing in tiny "hairs" with an ash-colored pencil. You can see what a great difference just that extension made in framing the eyes. The slight puffiness above the eyelid crease was diminished by using a khaki contour color contrasted with a pink eyelid color and a nude pink highlighter. A smudge of the same khaki color was placed along the roots of the last half of her lower lashes. The lashes were separated and made to look longer and thicker with mascara. A trace of white eyeshadow pencil on the inside lower rim of the eye opened the eye even more.

A warm pink powder rouge brushed onto the cheekbone and blended down into a deeper pinky-brown cheek contour accentuated Kandice's bone structure. A scant dusting of pink, highly pearlized powder highlighted the crest of her cheekbones, making them look higher.

Her lips were balanced by using a maroon lip pencil. The upper lip was defined following the natural lip line. The bottom lip was made less full by placing the lipliner within the lips rather than along the natural lip line, especially at the corners. The lips were then filled in with a pink lipstick/clear gloss combination.

To heighten the sculptured look of Kandice's face, the crease above the chin was shadowed with contour.

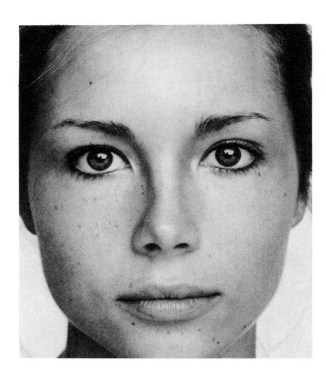

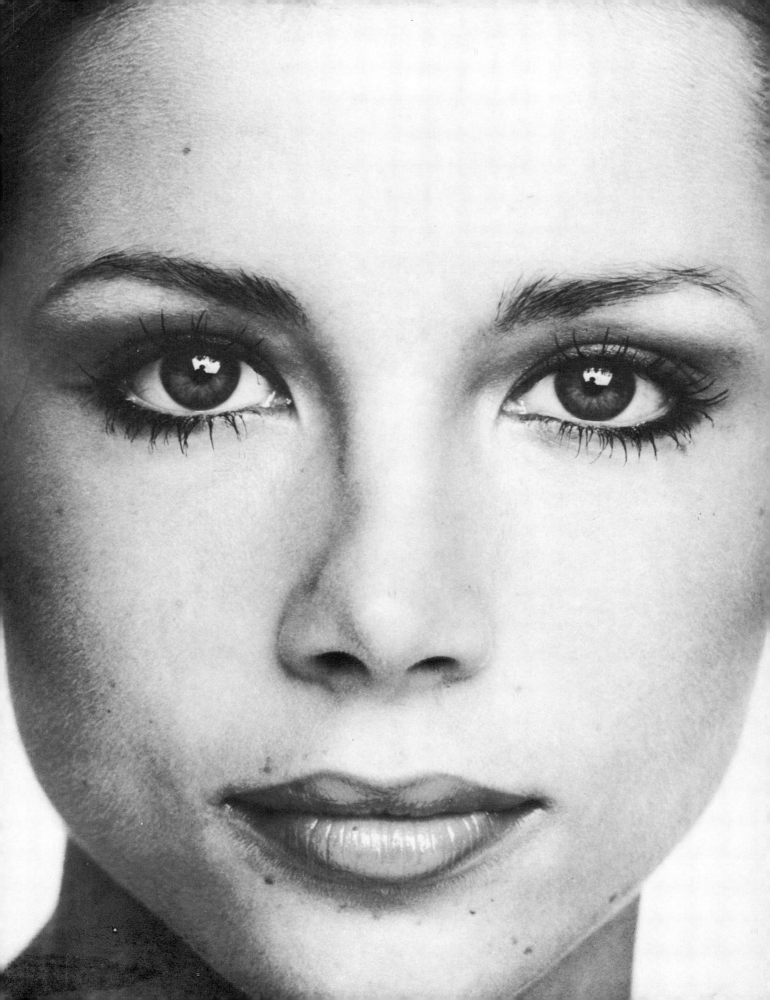

BARBARA

Barbara's fresh young look is intensified by clarifying her features. A film of liquid foundation was blended on, followed by a dusting of translucent powder. The area between the brows and the lashes was expanded by blending an off-white powder shadow from the brows down to where a warm brown contour color corrected the slight puffiness above the natural crease of the eyelid. A frosted opal color was applied to the lid to emphasize the lovely almond shape of the eyes. A smudgeline of charcoal soft eyeshadow pencil was placed along both the upper and lower lids. Black eyeshadow pencil was applied to the upper inside rim for clarification. Mascara was brushed on twice to create greater length and thickness.

The nostrils were defined with contour so that the tip of the nose had more of a chiseled look, and the chin was also defined with contour, creating a slight cleft. The cheeks were highlighted with a pearlized orangey-brown cream cheek color and defined with a warm brown contour color. The lips were balanced and defined with a light-brown lipliner, and then the lips were filled in with a warm brownish orange lipgloss/lipstick combination.

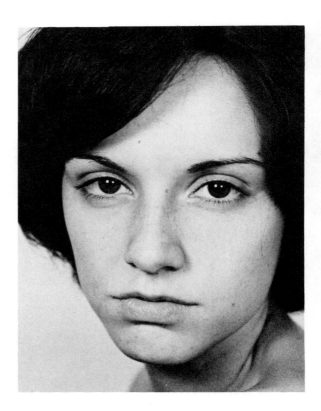

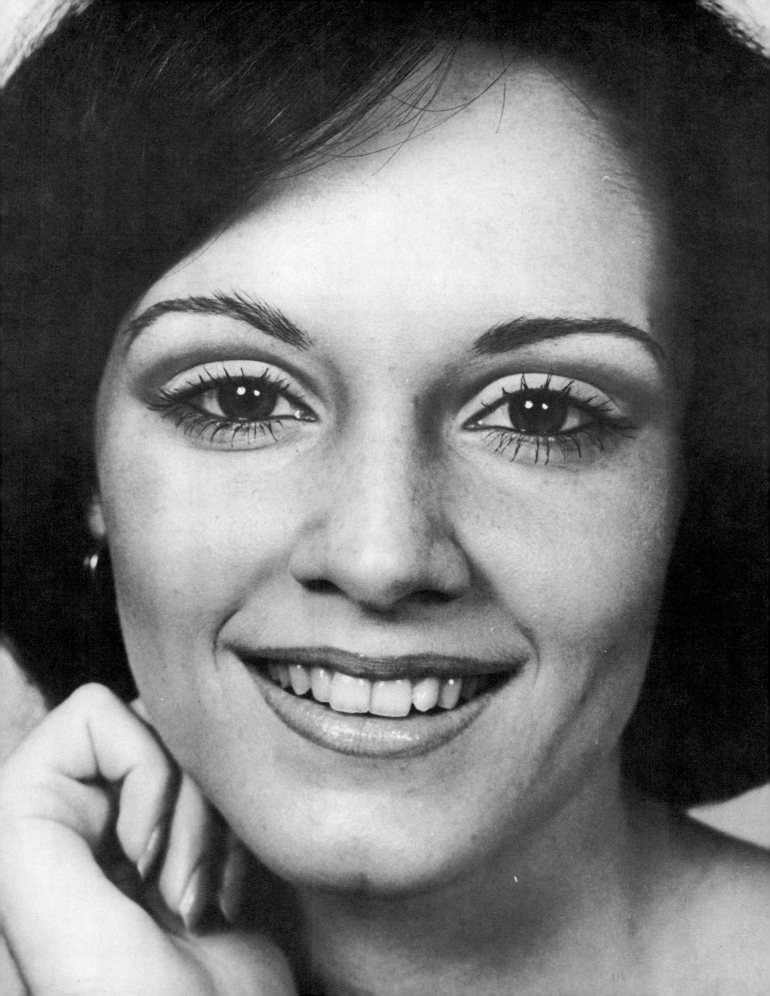

JOLINDA

Jolinda's fiery good looks were easily emphasized by defining her features. The first step was to create an even facial tone by applying whipped cream foundation and powder to achieve a matte effect. The eye area was intensified with a rust-colored eye contour, a golden peach eyelid color, and a gold pearl highlight. To expand the area just below the beginning of the brow, a white super highlight was applied, which gives the appearance of a higher brow. The inside rims of the lids were lined with charcoal eye pencil, and Jolinda's lashes were emphasized by applying mascara with thickener.

The roundness of Jolinda's face was de-emphasized by brushing her temples and the area beneath the cheekbone with a warm brown contour color. This shadowing created hollows which give the illusion of a more dramatic bone structure. The cheekbone was further accentuated by blending a highlighter along the very crest of the bone.

Jolinda's lips were more clearly defined by outlining with a red pencil, then filling in with a red lipstick and dotting the middle of each lip with a touch of red lipgloss.

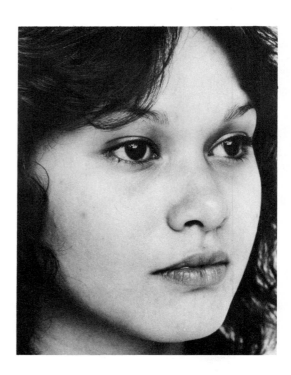

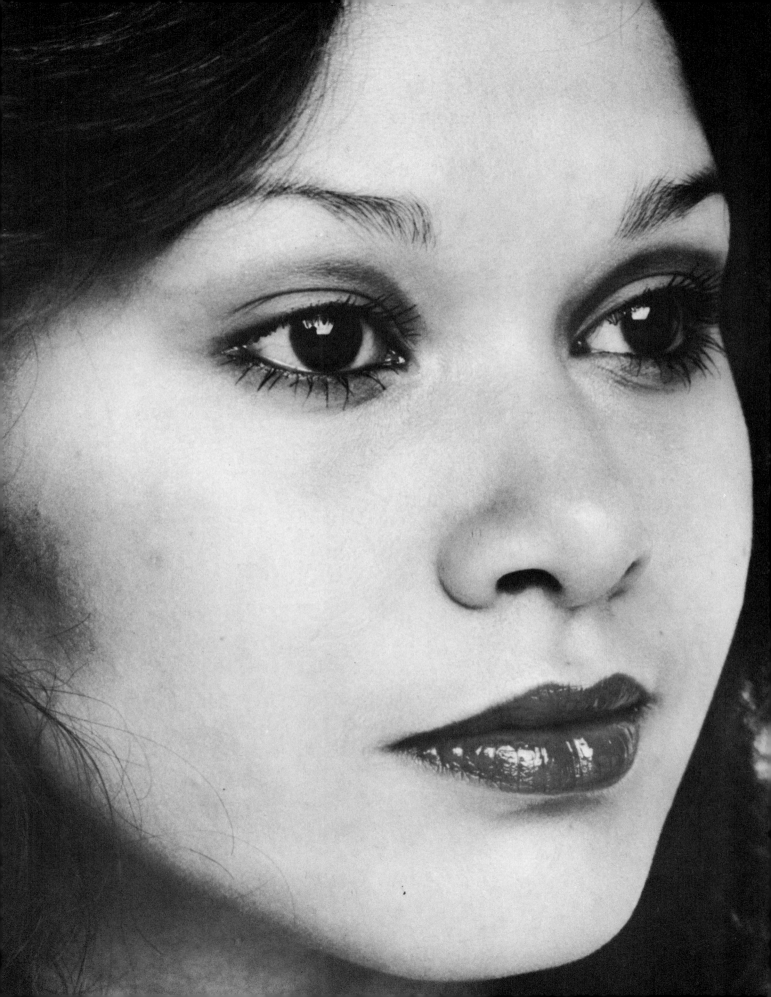

APPENDIX

I am not a believer in charts. It's hard to tell someone what colors to select because what I describe as coral or teal or bright red may mean something altogether different to you. It's also difficult to select colors for someone unless you actually see that someone. I have no way of knowing what shade of red hair you have, or how pale your pale complexion is.

Nevertheless, I want to give you general guidelines, and the only way I can do that is to name actual items because, as previously mentioned, "red" is meaningless unless we both have the same shade of red in mind.

In an effort to be more explicit, I have prepared the following charts using actual ON STAGE products, because these are the ones with which I am most familiar. Go to one of the ON STAGE sources (a complete listing follows) and look at the colors so that you can visualize the shades I recommend. Then, if you like, duplicate these colors in whichever line of cosmetics you use.

Do remember two very important things. First, my suggestions are very broad; when I say blonde, blue eyes, fair skin, that covers a **wide** spectrum, so be flexible. Second, the lifeblood of any good cosmetic line is its fashionability, its being up to date with fashion trends. Colors therefore change, and names change, too. So if the color I mention in the chart has been discontinued, allow the trained professional behind the counter to suggest another. Their advice is certain to be accurate . . . you're standing right in front of them!

ON STAGE POWDER EYE COLOR TRIOS

		Blue Eyes	Green Eyes	Hazel/Brown Eyes	Dark Brown Eyes
	BLONDE HAIR				
lid		Sapphire	Moss	Violet	Opal
contour		Slate	Cinnamon	Burlap	Khaki
highlight		Pink	Cream	Teal	Cream
	LIGHT BROWN HAIR				
lid		Brown	Rust	Teal	Adriatic
contour		Windsor	Khaki	Grey Brown	Slate
highlight		Nude Pink	Cream	White	Nude Pink
	DARK BROWN HAIR				
lid		Burlap	Rose	Jade	Claypot
contour		Grey Brown	Grey Brown	Khaki	Cinnamon
highlight		Cream	Pink	Yellow	Pink
	BLACK HAIR				
lid		Putty	Emerald	Moss	Paprika
contour		Wedgewood	Charcoal Brown	Slate	Brick
highlight		White	Lime	Pink	Brown
	GREY HAIR				
lid		Lavender	Opal	Blue	Lilac
contour		Slate	Ocean	Slate	Slate
highlight		Nude Pink	White	Cream	Pink
	RED HAIR				
lid		Emerald	Copper	Camel	Pink
contour		Cinnamon	Khaki	Khaki	Rust
highlight		Cream	Topaz	Cream	White

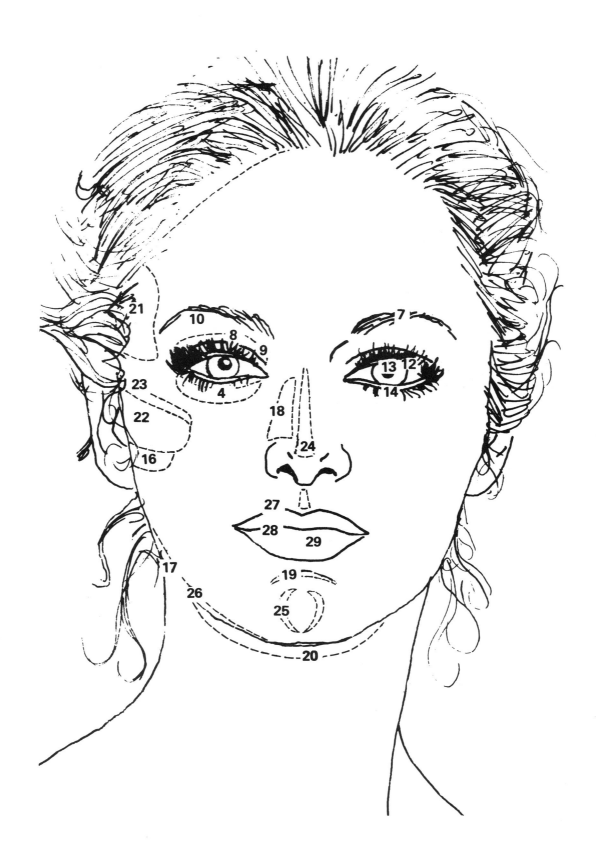

	ZONE	PRODUCT		TOOL
1	Cleanser	☐ Floataway ☐ Milk Float ☐ Eye Make-Up Remover		☐ Fingertips ☐ Cotton Wad
2	Skin Toner	☐ Astringent ☐ Freshener		☐ Cotton Wad
3	Moisture Cream	☐ Underbase ☐ Enriched		☐ Fingertips
4	Undereye/Blemish	☐ Touch		☐ Q-Tip
5	Foundation	☐ Liquid	☐ Mousse	☐ Dry Foam Sponge
6	Translucent Powder	☐ Loose ☐ Frosted	☐ Pressed	☐ Powder Brush
7	Brow Color	☐ Powder	☐ Pencil	☐ #4 Wedge Brush Pencil
8	Eye Contour	☐ Powder	☐ Cream	☐ #4 Wedge Brush ☐ Fluff Brush
9	Eyelid	☐ Powder	☐ Cream	☐ #8 Brush ☐ #6 Brush
10	Eye Highlight	☐ Powder	☐ Cream	☐ #1 Brush ☐ #6 Brush
11	Eye Liner	☐ Cake	☐ Fattie	☐ #00 Brush
12	Mascara	☐ Fattie	☐ 7" Pencil	☐ Fattie ☐ 7" Pencil
13	Upper Inside Eye Rim	☐ Fattie	☐ 7" Pencil	☐ Fattie ☐ 7" Pencil
14	Lower Inside Eye Rim	☐ Brown ☐ Waterp.	☐ Black ☐ Thick.	☐ Brush Wand
15	Lashes	☐ Brown	☐ Black	☐ Tweezer
16	Cheek Contour	☐ Powder	☐ Cream	☐ Contour Brush
17	Jaw Contour	☐ Powder	☐ Cream	☐ #10 Brush ☐ Contour Brush
18	Nose Contour	☐ Powder	☐ Cream	☐ #10 Brush
19	Chin Contour	☐ Powder	☐ Cream	☐ #10 Brush
20	Under Chin Contour	☐ Powder	☐ Cream	☐ Contour Brush
21	Temple Contour	☐ Powder	☐ Cream	☐ Contour Brush
22	Cheek Color	☐ Powder	☐ Cream	☐ Rouge Brush
23	Cheek Highlight	☐ Powder	☐ Cream	☐ #6 Brush
24	Nose Highlight	☐ Powder	☐ Cream	☐ #1 Brush
25	Chin Highlight	☐ Powder	☐ Cream	☐ #1 Brush
26	Jaw Highlight	☐ Powder	☐ Cream	☐ #10 Brush
27	Lip Outline	☐ Pencil	☐ Lipstick	☐ Lipliner ☐ Lip Brush
28	Lip Color	☐ Lipstick	☐ Lip Gloss	☐ Lip Brush
29	Lip Highlight	☐ Lip Gloss	☐ Dust	☐ Lip Brush

FOUNDATION, LIPSTICK, LIPGLOSS, & CHEEK COLOR HARMONIES

	Blonde		Brunette		Black		Grey/Salt & Pepper		Auburn/Red	
	Earthtones	Rose/Mauve	Earthtones	Rose/Mauve	Earthtones	Rose/Mauve	Earthtones	Rose/Mauve	Earthtones	Rose/Mauve
FOR LIGHT COMPLEXION: BISQUE OR SAND FOUNDATION										
Lipstick	Westside	Sutton Pl.	Bklyn	Soho	Bronx	Sutton Pl.	7th Ave.	West 4th	7th Ave.	42nd St.
Lipstick & Lip Gloss Combination	C.P.W. & Glace	125th St. & Watermelon	55th St. & Bronze	Bklyn & Glorioso	Madison Ave. & Terracotta	West 4th St. & Cattail	Bronx & Clear	Queens & Glace	Murray Hill & Watermelon	125th St. & Malta
Lip Gloss (with no lipstick)	Bronze	Cattail	Walnut	Orange	Malta	Bronze	Watermelon	Bronze	Cattail	
Powder Rouge	Adobefrost	Pink	Peachfrost	Mocha	Adobefrost	Pink	Adobefrost	Pink	Peachfrost	Mocha
Creme Rouge	Bronze	Mocha	Bronzefrost	Rosefrost	Bronzefrost	Rose	Bronze	Mochafrost	Bronze	Rose
FOR MEDIUM COMPLEXIONS: TAWNY OR PEACH FOUNDATION										
Lipstick	Park Ave.	42nd St.	Chelsea	125th St.	Murray Hill	Village	Park Ave.	42nd St.	Chelsea	125th St.
Lipstick & Lip Gloss Combination	7th Ave. & Glorioso	Queens & Malta	Park Ave. & Clear	Village & Glorioso	Chelsea & Walnut	E. 59th St. & Glace	Bklyn & Clear	8th St. & Red	West Side & Walnut	34th St. & Glace
Lip Gloss (with no lipstick)	Orange	Red	Ariel	Malta	Ariel	Cordovan	Ariel	Cattail	Orange	Red
Powder Rouge	Peach	Mocha	Peach	Mocha	Orange	Mocha	Peach	Mocha	Peach	Dark Mocha
Creme Rouge	Bronzefrost	Mochafrost	Bronze	Rose	Bronze	Rosefrost	Bronzefrost	Rose	Chili	Rosefrost
FOR TAN COMPLEXIONS: HONEY, AMBER OR BRONZE FOUNDATION										
Lipstick	Bronx	Village	Bronx	B'dway	C.P.W.	125th St.	Bklyn	8th St.	C.P.W.	Park Ave.
Lipstick & Lip Gloss Combination	Murray Hill & Walnut	Midtown & Cattail	55th St. & Clear	E. 59th St. & Cattail	Bronx & Ariel	Midtown & Mahogany	C.P.W. & Glace	34th St. & Watermelon	55th St. & Ariel	Bklyn & Malta
Lip Gloss (with no lipstick)	Terracotta	Mahogany	Glorioso	Cordovan	Terracotta	Mahogany	Glorioso	Red	Walnut	Mahogany
Powder Rouge	Orange	Pinkfrost	Brickfrost	Raspberryfrost	Brickfrost	Raspberryfrost	Orange	Pinkfrost	Orange	Raspberryfrost
Creme Rouge	Chili	Rose	Chili	Autumn Elm	Autumn Beech	Autumn Maple	Bronze	Red	Autumn Beech	Autumn Elm
FOR BLACK COMPLEXIONS: CHESTNUT, COCO, CAFE OR EXPRESSO FOUNDATIONS										
Lipstick			Madison Ave.	Midtown	Bronx	125th St.	Park Ave.	42nd St.	55th St.	Midtown
Lipstick & Lip Gloss Combination			Murray Hill & Clear	34th St. & Malta	Murray Hill & Ariel	Midtown & Mahogany	Madison Ave. & Terracotta	125th St. & Cattail	Bronx & Walnut	8th St. & Red
Lip Gloss (with no lipstick)			Ariel	Cordovan	Walnut	Mahogany	Terracotta	Red	Ariel	Malta
Powder Rouge			Peach	Raspberryfrost	Brickfrost	Red	Brickfrost	Raspberryfrost	Brickfrost	Red
Creme Rouge			Chili	Red	Chili	Autumn Elm	Chili	Red	Autumn Maple	Autumn Elm
FOR ORIENTAL COMPLEXIONS: TAWNY AND HONEY FOUNDATIONS										
Lipstick					Park Ave.	Village	Bklyn	Soho		
Lipstick & Lip Gloss Combination					55th St. & Walnut	125th St. & Cattail	Bronx & Ariel	42nd St. & Red		
Lip Gloss (with no lipstick)					Glorioso	Cordovan	Walnut	Malta		
Powder Rouge					Peach	Raspberryfrost	Orange	Mocha		
Creme Rouge					Chili	Autumn Elm	Bronze	Rose		

The following is a list of places where ON STAGE make-up may be purchased.

ON STAGE Accounts

ALABAMA
Auburn: Frieta's Finishing School
Birminghan: Mara Sandhaus
Cullman: Plaza Beauty Salon
Tuscaloosa: The Iron Horse

ARIZONA
Scottsdale: Armando Hair Design Facial Designs

CALIFORNIA
Anaheim: Barbizon School
Beverly Hills: M. G. Westmore, Cosmetic Center, Quido Umberto
Camarillo: Facial Frame
Carson: The Nail Shop
Cerritos: Vogue Hair Design
Costa Mesa: Hair Factory
Escondido: House of Lords
Freemont: Lewis & Co. Hair Design
Gilrow: Midge's Beauty Salon
Granada Hills: Wayne's Mod Squad
Hollywood: Basic Boutique
Irvine: Newport Academy of Modeling & Acting
Laguna Niguel: Hair Place
Lake Tahoe: Pazazz
Lakewood: Marty Harvey
Long Beach: Pygmalion Salon Lady Fingers
Los Alamitos: Barbizon School
Los Altos: Sumi
Los Angeles: Make-Up Center
Monterey: Laurie Andreone
Northridge: Hair Grove
Redondo Beach: Dino Brisgnano Hair and Nails
San Diego: Hair Shop, Headliners Salon of Hair, Scissors Society
San Francisco: Hair Doctor, Mister Lee
San Jose: San Jose City College
San Marino: Gates of Spain
San Mateo: Face Place, Master Lee Hair Stylist
San Rafael: Shy Looks, Suz Inc.
Santa Rosa: Antoinette's Fingers and Nails
Solano Beach: The Touch
Spring Valley: Di Maris Hair Studio
Torrance: Ramone Gallegos, Tates International
Van Nuys: Hairdressers
Vista: Nailworks
Westwood: The Make-Up Center of California, The Nail Garden

COLORADO
Fort Collins: Elan

CONNECTICUT
Bridgeport: Creative Co., Inc.
Hamden: Frances K. Merlowe
Manchester: Tres Chic Salon
New London: Jon Roberto
Stamford: HRH Hairdressers
Waterbury: Shears Gallery
Watertown: Jonathans Coiffures
Westport: Body Scents of Lauren

DELAWARE
Wilmington: Mrs. Audrey Diker, The Lock Smythe

DISTRICT OF COLUMBIA
Washington, D.C.: Hair Designers, The Make-Up Center, The Make-Up Center/Georgetown

FLORIDA
Bal Harbor: Balmoral Boutique
Boca Raton: About Faces Inc.
Cape Coral: New York Academy of Modeling
Coral Gables: Ugo di Roma
Fort Lauderdale: Christine Valmy Skin Care Center
Hollywood: Face Graffitti, Hair Connection
Jacksonville: Hair Designers of Jacksonville
Key West: The Hair People
Miami: Burdines (Beauty Salon), The Make-Up Center of Florida, Penthouse Coiffures, Ugo di Roma
Winter Park: Martie Schmidt

GEORGIA
Albany: Beauty Lounge & Boutique
Millen: Louise Lane

HAWAII
Honolulu: Hale O'Nails, The Make-Up Center/Hawaii, Maurice Damien, Tsuki's Hairstylist
Koloa/Kauai: Island Beauties

ILLINOIS
Chicago: J. Gordon Designs, United Airlines
Flossmoor: Jan Deingott Ent.
Glenview: T. Andre Designs
Homewood: Cosmetic Connection
Oak Park: Essence

INDIANA
Indianapolis: L. S. Ayres & Co., The Bobbs Merrill
   Co., Inc., Optical Fashions
South Bend: Ranas Hair Fashions

KANSAS
Hutchinson: The New Hayden's
Parsons: Dana Richardson
Wichita: Patricia Stevens School

KENTUCKY
Lexington: Kentucky Business College

LOUISIANA
New Orleans: Let's Face It
Shreveport: The Hair Shapers, Connie Harvey

MARYLAND
Baltimore: Barbizon School, Coco & Buff,
   Cut-Above
Bethesda: Miva Cosmetic Care
Chevy Chase: Barbizon School, Sarita's Beauty
   Clinic
Crofton: Robert Andrew of Crofton
Forestville: Kay's Hairmate
Gaithersburg: Kumiko's
Laurel: Kay's Kut & Kurl
North Bethesda: Rainbow Hair Designers
Pikesville: Esthetique Inc., Natural Beauty
Rockville: Face Place
Silver Spring: Headlines
Wheaton: Amy of Denmark

MASSACHUSETTS
Newton Center: Jane Aransky
Saugus: Narcissus
West Roxbury: Lords and Ladys Hair Salon

MICHIGAN
Detroit: Margie's Make-Up Specialty Shop
Flint: Evelyn Angel Salon
Jackson: Evaughn Rainey
Southfield: Visage

MINNESOTA
Minneapolis: Carole Belle, Lowthian School,
   Dorothy Lundstrom

MISSOURI
Florissani: Show Girl Nails
Kansas City: Pierre Brandli

NEBRASKA
Omaha: Patricia Stevens School

NEVADA
Las Vegas: Caesar's Palace Spa

NEW JERSEY
Atlantic City: Cricket & Co.
Cherry Hill: Clinique de Beaute
Clifton: Golda Jewell Beauty Salon
Fanwood: Skin Spa at Anton's
Fort Lee: The Nail Sensation, Women's World
Franklin Lakes: The Make-Up Center of New Jersey
Garfield: Salon Di Car
Hackensack: Barbara's Golden Scissors, Charm
   Beauty Salon, Richard Roberts
Hackettstown: Kerrs Pharmacy
Highland Park: Hair Fashions by Marta
Irvington: Salon de Leon
Jersey City: Mimmo Anton Salon
Margate: Salon Du Jour
Millburn: Nails Naturally
Montclair: Barbizon School
North Bergen: Grasshopper
Nutley: The Better Look
Oakland: A Cut Above
Palisades Park: Joanne Montenegro
Paramus: Barbizon School
Pompton Lakes: Plaza Hair Stylists
Princeton: Iris
Ridgefield: Hair Sensation
Ridgewood: Magic Touch Beauty Salon, Sealfons
   Specialty Shop
Rochelle Park: He & She
Toms River: Vicki's Make-Up Salon
Upper Montclair: Jon Rinaldi, Just Nails
West New York: Face Design
Woodridge: Beauty Forum, Rita Waldron (Peter's
   Beauty Salon)

NEW MEXICO
Albuquerque: Aquarius, Boutique of Beauty

NEW YORK

Albany: Biogenic Skin Care Center, Les Chiseaux

Albertson: Ultissima Haircutters

Babylon: Barbizon School

Bronx: Luigi of Italy

Brooklyn: Brandon Scott

Buffalo: John Robert Powers School

Clifton Park: Hair 2000, Inc.

Floral Park: Pourans Beauty and Boutique

Hicksville: Berreley School

Merrick: Maximus

New York: Bayardo Baredda, Essence of Beauty, Fashion Models, International Top Models, The Make-Up Center, Monica Pinnock, James Santa, Inc., Skin Clinic, Clive Summers, Inc.

Poughkeepsie: Bruno & Co., Trendsetter

Rego Park: Yolas Pamper People

Rochester: Upstate Careers (John Robert)

Rosalyn: Westwood Pharmacy

Salt Point: Cromwell Beauty Shoppe

Syracuse: Headlines, Umberto

Tewksbury: Shear Sex

Wappinger Falls: Mr. John Leonard

Westbury: Vista East Coiffures

White Plains: The Berkeley School

NORTH CAROLINA

Ashville: Creative Hair Design, Faces & Nails Ltd.

Burlington: Nails & Lash Boutique

Charlotte: American Business & Fashion Institute, Nails by the Finishing Touch

Gastonia: Nail Factory

Greensboro: The Difference Inc., Hair Care Center, Jeannie & Judy's Make-Up Center

Hendersonville: C'est Ca Cie Salons

Raleigh: John Robert Powers School

Shelby: Uptown Connection

OHIO

Akron: Bon Chic

Alliance: Patti Schaefer

Bedford: The Hair Hut

Canton: Ron Karl Hairstylists

Cincinnati: Hair Surgeon, Inc., The Nail Box, Stratford School of Fashion

Cleveland: Dorian Leigh Model Agency, Right Faces, Inc.

Columbus: The Hair Hunters, Wright Modeling Agency

Fairfield: Skin Deep, Southern Ohio College

Kirtland: Raun Hairdressers

Marion: Fantastique Salon

Painesville: Lady's First

Youngstown: The Beauty Corner

OKLAHOMA

Oklahoma City: Sonny's of Quail Creek

Shawnee: Joy's Hair Fashions

Sulfur: Sunshine Co.

OREGON

Eugene: Complexions, Robert's Townhouse

Lake Oswego: Heads Up

Portland: Marlene Frazel, Hickox & Friends, The Make-Up Center (Faces Unlimited)

PENNSYLVANIA

Altoona: Carol & Sandi's Beauty Salon

Bethel Park: Marian's Hair & Skin Care Salon

Carnegie: A Nu U

Center Valley: Ann M. Hirsch

Charleroi: Miller's

Emmaus: Jan Nagy

Jenkintown: Fabulous Face

Latrobe: Kurlique

McMurray: Stephen's Hairgraphics

Media: Skin Deep Beauty Clinic

New Hope: Queen of Sheba

Pittsburgh: Barranti's, Cosmetics by Lynn, Intriques, Kut & Kurl Beauty Bar, Leslie & Co., The Make-Up Center of Pittsburgh, Puccini's, Solomon's of Pittsburgh, Joseph de Stefino, Stephen's Hairgraphics, Super Hair Salon

Sharon: Cheena's World

Squirrel Hill: Philip Pelusi

Stroudsburg: Finishing Touch

Wyncote: Nails Unlimited

RHODE ISLAND

Cranston: Filomena's Hair Care Center, Transformation Ltd.

Newport: Ram's Head Inc.

Pawtucket: Ann Corbett

SOUTH CAROLINA

Camden: Guys & Dolls Beauty Shop

Charleston: Sandra Dee's, Fountain of Youth

Columbia: Ruth Ann Collins Modeling Studio, Fashion Merchandising, Make-Up Center, Ltd., Mille Lewis Studio, Kenneth Shuler's School

Florence: Studio One

Greenville: He & Me Hair Styles, Millie Lewis Studio

Hartsville: Holland House

Hilton Head Island: Millie Lewis Studio

Myrtle Beach: Costa Brava

Rock Hill: Village Square Salon

SOUTH DAKOTA
Sioux Falls: Nettleton College

TENNESSEE
Memphis: Patricia Stevens School
Nashville: Adam & Eve Salon

TEXAS
Alpine: Ladybug & Hair Co.
Beaumont: Up Your Alley Beauty
Conroe: Cin Bec Studio
Corpus Christi: McLaughlin's Adjunct
Dallas: Aesthetician's International, Inc., Coalesce
El Paso: Mannequin Manor
Fort Worth: Gary Martin Enterprises, The Shoppe
Galveston: Summitt Hair Art Studio
Higgins: House of Beauty
Houston: Cosmetique Ltd., Foley's Department Store
Kileen: Foxy Lady, Goldfinger's Hair Fashion
Kirbyville: Mary's House of Beauty
Lakehills: Cutaway
Lamesa: Teresa's Hairacy
Lubbock: The Gazebo Salon
Midland: The Headquarters
San Angelo: Act I, The Rage

UTAH
Provo: Career College of Beauty
Salt Lake City: Career Culture Center, McCarty Casting, Mr. Roberts Hair Fashions

VIRGINIA
Burke: Let's Make-Up
McLean: Hair Alive
Springfield: Kirk Sharon, Kircare Consultants
Richmond: Charles B. Baum
Vienna: Nail Sculptor
Virginia Beach: Beautiful Nails, Models Inc.

WASHINGTON
Ellensburg: Headhunter
Seattle: Gene Jaurez Hair & Cosmetics, Robert Leonard Ltd., The Make-Up Center of Washington
Tacoma: Vogue Modeling and Finishing School

WEST VIRGINIA
Huntington: Huntington School of Beauty & Culture

PUERTO RICO
Carquas: Hair Connections
San Juan: Sammy's Modern

FRANCE
Paris: Dans un Jardin, Jean-Louis David, Galeries Lafayette, The Make-Up Center, Ingrid Millet, Printemps, Jean-Pierre Richard

HONDURAS
The Make-Up Center

ITALY
Milano: Cose
Roma: Sergio Valente

VENEZUELA
Caracas: The Make-Up Center
Chain stores (approx. 130) throughout Venezuela: Cadena de Perfumeria, Sarela, Cadena de Perfumeria, Ipasme, Cadena de Almacenes, Ipsfa, Proveedu la Ciudad Universitaria, Cadena de Perfumerias mas por Menos, Cadena Dabuky en Maracay y Valencia, Cadena Dalmont en Valencia, Cadena Cooperativa Auyantepuy